BODY & SOUL

Karen Smith was a dancer with the Royal Ballet, London Festival Ballet and London City Ballet until she broke her neck in a car accident leaving her paralysed. Once able to walk again, her recovery assisted by the benefits of complementary medicine, she embarked on various training courses. Karen subsequently qualified as a reflexologist, masseuse and aromatherapist all of which she now teaches. As well as having a busy complementary practice in London, she teaches ballet and pilates practice.

For Sophie
with love
from
Karen

BODY & SOUL

A woman's guide to staying young

KAREN SMITH

Foreword by Maureen Lipman

KYLE CATHIE LIMITED

Acknowledgements

I would like to thank the following for their help and advice:

Roger Groos DHM, RCT, MCIA, BSc; Gerard Dooley BDS, NUI; Andrew Chevallier, FNIMH; Brian Butler BA, DO; The Bach Centre; Lotte Berk; Dreas Reyneke; Peter van Minnen.

I would also like to thank Ursula Hageli not only for being a wonderful model for the photographs but also for typing all my text!

My love and thanks to Tony for his encouragement and support during the writing of this book.

Finally I would like to thank the illustrator, David Downton, and the photographer, Katrina Lithgow; also Ruth Baldwin, my editors Candida Hall and Sophie Bessemer and everyone at Kyle Cathie Ltd who has contributed to *Body and Soul*.

First published in paperback 1998 by
Kyle Cathie Limited
20 Vauxhall Bridge Road, London SW1V 2SA

10 9 8 7 6 5 4 3 2 1

ISBN 1 85626 241 3

A Cataloguing in Publication record for this title is available from the British Library.

Designed by Ann Burnham
Cover designed by Sara-Jane Vere Nicoll
Edited by Candida Hall and Sophie Bessemer

The contents of this book are for information only and are intended to assist readers in identifying symptoms and conditions they may be experiencing. The book is not intended to be a substitute for taking proper medical advice and should not be relied upon in this way. Always consult a qualified doctor or health practitioner. The author and publisher cannot accept responsibility for illness arising out of the failure to seek medical advice from a doctor.

CONTENTS

This book is dedicated to Mum, Dad and all my family and friends who gave me support at a time when my own body and soul was at a very low ebb.

FOREWORD

by

Maureen Lipman

When I grew up in the 50s, the banned book in the house, that you stole at your peril and perused in the airing cupboard with a flashlight and a friend, was not *The Story of O* or *The Kama Sutra*, but a heavy, gloomily illustrated copy of *Pears Encyclopaedia of Health.*

Figuring out how the uterus could possibly fit into anywhere in your skinny pre-adolescent body or what on earth was the point of testicles suddenly popping in and out, was an endless source of rude delight but of very little real information. Anyway, the remedies remained constant in our house. Hot milk and butter (aargh!) for sore throats. Vic rubbed on the chest for – er – chestiness. Fenning's Powders for colds, Beecham's for flu, liver salts for stomach upsets and chicken soup for everything.

Over the intervening years I have formed a compulsive interest in alternative medicine and an open-minded attitude to suiting the treatment to the patient not just the general ailment. I will reach for an aspirin as fast as the next stressed person but I will also use the long-term healing properties of reflexology, shiatsu massage and herbal or homeopathic preventatives, often to beneficial effect. Perhaps women are particularly drawn to holistic medicine, since it involves feelings, emotions and intuition, rather than just chemical fact, but the proof of the power of mind and body interaction is so overwhelming now that we would be blind to ignore it.

With *Body and Soul*, Karen Smith has set out to write a comprehensive and clear laywoman's guide to the body's workings, weaknesses and needs. Simply, straightforwardly, she takes the curious, the fascinated and even the mild hypochondriacs like myself, through the effects of ageing, and changes of lifestyle on our systems, and exactly how we can improve our health.

This is a guide for your coffee table, your desk, your study – or even your airing cupboard if it makes you feel better.

INTRODUCTION

Good health and mobility is something we all take for granted during our younger years. I was no exception, and having been a ballet dancer for thirty years I accepted my physical capabilities without a second thought. Then came the night when fate took a hand, changing my life and my perceptions with it. One moment I was performing the lead role in a ballet performance and within two hours of curtain down I was in casualty paralysed from the neck down after a serious car accident. Luck, however, was on my side as today I am fully recovered, but it has been a slow process. Not only were there physiological problems but also emotional hurdles to overcome. My career ended, I had lost a part of my life for which I held a great passion and with it went my confidence and self esteem.

Complementary medicine has always fascinated me, so I adopted many of the therapies available to assist my recovery. My health improved so much that I decided a few years later to train in massage, anatomy and physiology, aromatherapy, reflexology and nutrition. I became engrossed in everything I learnt at seminars and lectures and soon realized that I could benefit others by passing on my newly acquired knowledge.

Once qualified and working in a clinic situation I became aware that many people were ignorant of their body's functions and had accepted their health problems might never change. They genuinely believed that feeling below average was the norm. It was this which prompted me to write a health book for women (although many sections will be suitable for men).

Women are usually more intuitive and generally more concerned about their health than men, maybe this is because our state of health affects our physical appearance, something which often concerns women more than men.

This book is intended to be used by women from forty to ninety nine, however it is never too early to care about one's health so the book is equally suitable for a younger woman. After all, prevention is cheaper than treatment.

I begin the book by discussing the ageing process, and the steps we can take to combat its effects. By the turn of the century more than half of the population will be over fifty. People are now living far longer than they did forty years ago. Just to take one example, England in the early 50s had 200 centenarians living – now there are almost 3,000.

To maintain good health it is vital that you understand more about the human body, it's functions, what can go wrong and some ways of helping. Illness is a war within the body therefore it is wise to learn about the enemy in order to cope with it. Conditions such as arthritis, heart attacks and osteoporosis, were not created by nature, but as a result of man's autonomy.

It is well known that what we endure emotionally affects our health quite significantly, therefore one of the best ways to look after the body is to reduce stress levels. Alternative therapies, no longer regarded as eccentric, are rapidly gaining approval from many orthodox practitioners and are a natural part of many people's lives. I hope that my overview of the different therapies and self help techniques you can do at home will encourage you to discover a method that really works for you.

In the prevention of illness and the maintenance of good health I do not ignore the benefits of exercise. Whatever your age, build and physical capability there is an exercise to suit you.

Inevitably the years and certain indulgences along the way will take their toll nutritionally within our bodies. As we mature our essential organs become less resilient, so we must learn to treat them with better care. My appraisal of women's health concludes with a practical guide to the important nutrients for life, and how our diet can supply them – the vitamins, minerals and herbs that can cleanse and detoxify our system. Good nutrition is not about denial but about moderation, balance and health awareness. It is the quality and enjoyment of life that matters – our body and health is a reflection of who we are.

Unlike so many conventional works on the subject, *Body and Soul* offers you choices at every stage. Use it as a reference guide or read it at leisure. You are what you eat, drink, breathe and think so good health is your best investment!

physiological factors

AGEING
- Why do we age
- Cells

BODY SYSTEMS
- Skeletal
- Neurological
- Endocrine
- Immune
- Lymphatic
- Digestive
- Urinary
- Cardiovascular
- Respiratory
- Reproductive
- Hair
- Skin
- Teeth
- Eyes

AGEING

part one

There are three types of age: chronological (ruled by the calendar); biological (instructed by the body's processes); psychological (how old one feels). It is the quality of an individual's life rather than the length which is important.

Ageing is a universal, inevitable, natural and genetic process. The one thing we all share is that we are born, grow to maturity and eventually we die. Ageing happens differently to everyone, not only in the way they age but also in the way they react to ageing. Flexibility of mind, body and spirit ultimately determines physical appearance and state of health, regardless of chronological age. We don't grow old, but we become old when we cease to grow and to adapt.

Relatively few people die of old age. Most die because as we age we lose our ability to adapt to change, the body being less efficient at coping with physical or environmental stress. Remarkably, the human body is self-repairing and self-maintaining. On a cellular level we are constantly undergoing replacement and repair, but the process slowly loses strength and pace, causing us to age. Why does this happen? There are many contributory factors, such as the effects of improper nutrition, environmental influences, exposure to toxins in the environment and in our food, exposure to sunlight, drugs and stress and lack of exercise.

Most of these are within our control. Nature has given us the ability to live a healthy and productive life, but the chances of disease and early ageing are often increased by our lifestyle. By making changes now to our way of living, we can reduce the chance of illness in later life, no matter how old we are.

GROW OLD GRACEFULLY

There is no need to inflict ageing on yourself and so 'become' old. Be comfortable with growing older as a natural part of life and stay young mentally.

WHY DO WE AGE?

There are three main factors responsible for ageing:

Genes Although not yet proven, it is thought that one or more of our genes actually dictates cellular ageing within the nucleus (core) of the cell, or that certain genes are either suppressed or extracted during the normal process of living.

Damage Naturally occurring chemical reactions within the body begin to produce a number of irreversible defects in molecules. These can be due to viruses, trauma, free radicals and pollution. With ageing, the body's natural repair processes become less effective, which can then cause system failure.

Imbalance With age the brain, endocrine and immune systems begin to function less efficiently. Our internal body clocks slow down, decreasing the production of important hormones. The immune system weakens, lowering our resistance to infection, and the degeneration of the brain can affect the functioning of the complex nervous system. However, these systems may age at different rates, producing an imbalance among the systems as well as a reduction in effectiveness within each one. It is when this occurs that we become prone to many degenerative conditions such as arthritis, osteoporosis and heart disease. Research, however, has shown that in some so-called less-developed countries, where the diet consists mainly of natural foods such as fish, grains and fruit, the inhabitants not only live longer but they are rarely prone to western degenerative diseases. Nutrition may therefore play a very important part in longevity.

THE CELLS

The cell is the smallest basic structural unit in the body. We each consist of billions of these cells, integrated structurally and functionally to perform complex physiological life assignments.

Different types of cell are designated for specific tasks such as transporting oxygen, engulfing and digesting harmful bacteria, producing hormones and conducting electro-chemical messages from the nervous tissue throughout the body. There are also connective tissue cells which include fat cells, cells that form cartilage and fibrous and elastic tissues which bind the body together, and muscle cells. The cell is continuously moving, growing and reproducing. Sending and receiving messages from the outside, it is the source of our constant life energy and is responsible for the body's youthfulness and longevity. A cell's memory records its past experiences, but if the memories are lost cellular functions become impaired. A perfect memory in a cell would lead to immortality.

CELLULAR BREAKDOWN

Because the cell is so intricate it can easily be disturbed, which may cause its entire function to be seriously damaged. When you think of the vast number of cells there are in the body, it becomes apparent that degeneration and ageing begin as a result of cellular breakdown. The ageing of the cells determines our biological age; our chronological age is only a small share of the ageing process. By the time you reach 70 your cells will look unique, echoing your experiences both mentally and physically.

During a normal lifetime we replace our cells approximately eight times, with the exception of those in the nervous system which are very slow to regenerate. With time and continued use, the cells become littered with each biological drama, recording it in the form of toxic debris. This causes clogged pigments, cross-linked molecules and damaged DNA. The result is ageing.

Another reason why cells age is that the mitochondria (the cells' energy conversion factories) wear out. According to James E. Flemming of the Linus Pauling Institute in the USA, it is these mitochondria which are really the site of primary lesions which occur during ageing because that is where all the damage takes place.

Cell division occurs frequently throughout life in the skin, intestines and immune system, and occasionally in the kidneys and liver whose processes they are able to rejuvenate. The liver is the only organ that has the ability to regenerate itself in many cases. However, cardiac cells, neurones (nerve cells) and some smooth muscle cells never divide. In the end damage to the mitochondria in the non-dividing cells leads to an insufficient production of chemical energy to drive all the reactions that are needed for formal cell function. The cells simply run down as any machine would.

DAMAGE TO DNA

DNA has remained almost the same for 600 million years. It is unique in that it can reproduce itself. It can, however, become damaged by free radicals as a result of exposure to toxins, including those found in cigarettes, alcohol, drugs and caffeine. If the damage is not too great, it may be self-repairing; if it is serious, future generations of cells will become ruined.

DNA

DNA (deoxyribonucleic acid) is the hereditary gene material in each cell. It is the master molecule of all bodily functions and is our own personal genetic coding. It specifies an individual's height, eye, hair and skin colour, blood tissue type and general physiological make-up. Without DNA no life would exist on earth. Together with its messenger RNA (ribonucleic acid), DNA carries the coded genetic instructions in the cells. It acts as a sequence for RNA manufacture, providing the coding instructions necessary for protein synthesis (the process by which the body unlocks amino acids from proteins in order to make use of them). Damage to DNA is now accepted as a major cause of ageing.

Does the secret lie in our genes?

Genes are the basic units of genetic material carried at a particular area in our chromosomes, threadlike structures in the nucleus of each cell. They are relatively simple cogs in the incredibly sophisticated machinery of our bodies. If one of these cogs goes wrong it can have far-reaching effects and genetic desease can result.

Although genetic conditions can be influenced by diet, weight and lifestyle, as many as a dozen genes may contribute towards our susceptibility to them.

Researchers such as Professor Tom Kirkwood of Manchester University suggest that a genetic defect could certainly give rise to premature ageing. Similar patterns of gene inheritance can give members of the same species comparable life spans. All the factors affecting ageing are unknown and probably differ between people – a long healthy life or lack of it could just be a result of good or bad luck in the genetic lottery.

FREE RADICALS

Free radicals are chemically reactive unstable molecules which the body has to handle on a daily basis. They are a secondary product from the continuous reactions within the body, so the most commonly found are oxygen free radicals. Generally, these FRs are necessary for the normal functioning of the metabolic processes and are helped by various enzymes, without which we would die.

When kept in control, free radicals are essential to the immune system, as the white blood cells use them to bond with and destroy invading bacteria and viruses. However, their volatile nature means they are easily destabilised. Inevitably, our ever-increasing pollution is cited as the main catalyst for this. Once set free, the FRs cause abnormal oxidization and havoc within the cells. Uncontrolled, they may increase the number of cancer cells and are known to have a detrimental effect on mobility, skin wrinkling, the build-up of cholesterol and progressive hardening of the veins and arteries, all of which contribute to premature ageing.

HOW GENES MAY AFFECT US

Our genetic makeup will influence the development of the following chronic diseases:

- **Coronary heart disease.**
- **Stroke.**
- **Diabetes.**
- **Cancer (most forms).**

RISK FACTORS

The primary threats to free radicals are:

- **Cigarette smoke.**
- **Traffic fumes.**
- **Radiation (from X-rays, nuclear power stations and electro-magnetic fields).**

BODY SYSTEMS

part two

There is an internal universe within the body. This section explains very simply how the body's different systems function, how they are inter-related, what can go wrong when there is an imbalance and the many ways to prevent and improve this.

When we think about ageing, we are likely to focus on our outward appearance. We accept that losing our sight a little and developing grey hairs and wrinkles could be part of the ageing process. However, misconception about the body's many functions and their influence on the ageing process can blind us to the true nature of ageing. It is the events taking place *inside* the body which are far deeper and more deceptive. Understanding the inevitable changes, both physical and emotional, that occur as we grow older will therefore enable us to cope with them more naturally.

Skeletal

FUNCTION

• The human skeletal system comprises 206 named bones and, together with the muscles and joints, is responsible for body movement.

• The skeleton also provides a protective framework for the internal organs and helps to manufacture vital blood cells.

• The most common disorders of the skeletal system are osteoporosis, osteoarthritis and rheumatoid arthritis.

Bone is a living tissue consisting of around 90 per cent calcium and other minerals. Its growth and renewal depend on two essential cells, osteoblasts and osteoclasts, which between them are responsible for the deposition of new bone or the absorption of old bone. The skeleton responds to pressure or physical stress, renewing itself many times during a lifetime. As we age, more bone is reabsorbed than formed, resulting in weakness, especially in the spine. In adults, bone mass formation is the end result of the interacting factors of heredity, exercise levels and hormonal and nutritional status.

Genetically women have less muscle bulk and bone mass than men and in later life, when levels of the hormone oestrogen fall, mineralization of the bone is impeded, restricting calcium absorption. This can lead to osteoporosis, particularly in post-menopausal women or in those who have undergone removal of the ovaries. Lack of collagen, the principal fibrous component of connective tissue, can also affect the deposition of calcium phosphate contributing to the loss of bone density.

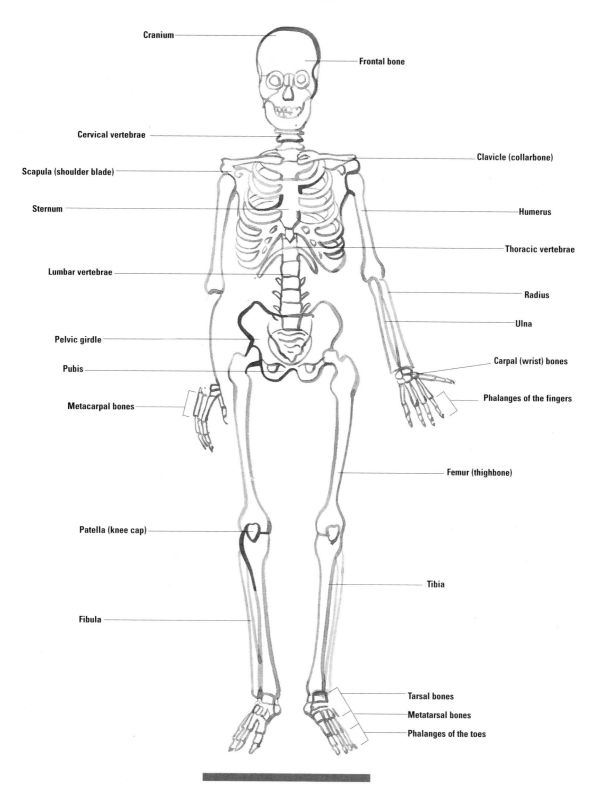

Cranium

Frontal bone

Cervical vertebrae

Clavicle (collarbone)

Scapula (shoulder blade)

Sternum

Humerus

Thoracic vertebrae

Lumbar vertebrae

Radius

Ulna

Pelvic girdle

Pubis

Carpal (wrist) bones

Metacarpal bones

Phalanges of the fingers

Femur (thighbone)

Patella (knee cap)

Tibia

Fibula

Tarsal bones

Metatarsal bones

Phalanges of the toes

RISK FACTORS

These include:

- Hereditary conditions.
- Early menopause (before 45).
- Early hysterectomy.
- Anorexia nervosa.
- Long-term use of steroids.
- Long-term smoking.
- Heavy alcohol intake.
- Poor nutrition.
- Lack of exercise.

WAYS OF HELPING OSTEOPOROSIS

- Increase exercise.
- Reduce protein intake.
- Stop smoking, reduce alcohol intake.
- Increase calcium intake, with magnesium and zinc for absorption.
- Increase vitamin D intake.
- Increase vitamin C to build calcium.
- Increase intake of boron.
- For natural oestrogen eat soya foods, fennel, celery, alfalfa, green and yellow vegetables and linseeds.
- HRT is sometimes prescribed.

OSTEOPOROSIS

Osteoporosis literally means 'porous bones' and, contrary to general belief, does not have to be an inevitable part of a woman's ageing process. There are many ways to prevent and help the condition.

Often there are no obvious symptoms, which is why it is sometimes referred to as the 'silent bone robber'. A fracture from a fall during a normal everyday activity is usually an early warning sign. Vulnerable areas for osteoporotic fractures are the wrist, hip, spinal vertebrae and femur. Curvature and shortening of the spine can be another sign, and in extreme cases the upper spinal vertebrae can form a dowager's hump if they become lodged.

Hysterectomy and ovary removal increase the rate of bone loss by causing a drop in oestrogen levels. Bone loss then steadily surpasses bone formation.

In addition to steroids, drugs such as Heparin (prescribed for heart disease and high blood pressure), diuretics, antacids and anti-convulsants can heighten bone loss. (It is important, though, not to stop taking any medication without first consulting your doctor.) Liver, endocrine and kidney disorders can alter blood calcium levels and bone metabolism. During pregnancy and lactation the body's calcium store can become depleted. According to Dr Ellen Grant in her book *Sexual Chemistry*, a chronic deficiency of zinc, which is essential for normal bone formation, is also a main cause of osteoporosis.

OSTEOARTHRITIS

Osteoarthritis is a degenerative disease of the joints. It is the most common type of arthritis and usually results from general wear and tear on the joints and cartilage. If there is a decrease in cartilage, friction occurs in the joints and a breakdown in collagen causes the ends of the bones to enlarge. The synovial fluid which normally lubricates the joints becomes stickier and less able to function. This in turn leads to joint restriction, swelling, pain and stiffness. It usually affects areas such as the hips, knees, hands and spine.

RHEUMATOID ARTHRITIS

Rheumatoid arthritis seems more common in women and can strike at any age, sometimes afflicting women as young as 25. Affected joints become swollen, painful and stiff. Structures around the joint may become inflamed, resulting in weakness of the ligaments, tendons and surrounding muscles and causing further pain and stiffness. Rheumatoid arthritis is thought to be an auto-immune disorder, the body's own natural defence against infection attacking its own tissues. Hormonal imbalances can affect the calcium balance, leading to arthritis. An impaired immune system, a poor diet and free radical damage can all pave the way for arthritis, so it is essential that your overall health regime is improved.

BACK PAIN

About 80 per cent of the population will suffer from back pain at some time and the problem is ever-increasing, causing the loss of millions of working days every year. The most common cause is muscle strain due to bad posture, overweight, weak abdominal muscles, or lifting or bending incorrectly. Correct spinal alignment allows a good balance of all the muscle groups around the spine giving it free support. Bad posture or a sedentary lifestyle can weaken the muscles leaving the skeleton inadequately supported. In turn this affects the joints and reduces the flexibility of muscles and ligaments.

Back pain can result from damage to nerves, discs or the spinal cord, nerve compression (sciatica), joint strain, deformities such as scoliosis, lordosis and kyphosis (types of spinal curvature), problems of ageing such as spondylosis (arthritic changes in the vertebrae) and spondylitis (vertebrae inflammation), osteoporosis (thinning of the bones) and inflammatory diseases like rheumatoid arthritis or scar tissue. Non-spinal causes of back pain can be kidney, gynaecological, gall bladder or colon problems, digestive ulcers, respiratory problems and even flu. There can also be emotional causes – our feelings can affect or manifest themselves in our backs in hunched shoulders or, if we are happy, 'walking tall'.

WAYS OF HELPING ARTHRITIS

- Exercise increases joint mobility – try yoga, swimming and stretching (see chapter four).
- Avoid weight gain which increases pressure on the joints.
- Reduce your fat and sugar intake.
- Take supplements of vitamin C and E, boron, calcium, magnesium and fish liver oils.
- Green-lipped mussel and shark cartilage contain mucopolysaccharides which assist the formation of cartilage.

WAYS OF HELPING BACK PAIN

These are a few of the treatments you could try (see chapter three for details):
- Physiotherapy.
- Rheumatology.
- Neurology.
- Orthopaedic treatment.
- Osteopathy.
- Chiropractic.
- Alexander technique.
- Massage.
- Reflexology.

Neurological

FUNCTION

The nervous system controls all that happens in the body. It is a complicated network consisting of:

- **The brain.**
- **The spinal cord.**
- **Various nerves.**

Together the brain and spinal cord form the central neurological (nervous) system whose role is to recieve sensory information from organs such as the eyes and ears and from receptors within the body. The brain consists of billions of nerve cells which are responsible for the transmission of messages to and from the brain. The spinal cord which extends from the brain stem then connects the brain to the body via a network of nerves. The central neurological system interprets the information received activating the appropriate motor response. All the nerves that are not part of the brain or spinal cord are part of the peripheral (near the surface) nervous system. Extending from the central nervous system to the muscles, skin, internal organs and glands are cranial nerves which come directly from the brain, and spinal nerves from the spinal cord. The two systems are linked in order to receive and deliver messages throughout the body. Nerve cells are very delicate and have limited potential for repair if they are damaged: nerve processes can repair, but not the cell nuclei. Spinal cord damage is permanent and peripheral nerves can be damaged by inflammation, infection, metabolic disorders and nutritional deficiencies. Three common disorders of the nervous system are Alzheimer's disease, Multiple sclerosis, and Parkinson's.

WAYS OF HELPING

- **Improve health and fitness to boost physical and mental wellbeing.**
- **Take Ginko Biloba to increase blood and oxygen flow to the brain.**
- **Research suggests supplements of vitamins E, C, beta-carotene and co-enzyme Q10 may help decrease the risk of developing Alzheimer's.**
- **B-complex and phosphatidyl choline help transmission of nerve impulses.**

ALZHEIMER'S DISEASE

Alzheimer's disease involves a progressive degeneration of the nerve cells in and subsequent shrinkage of the brain and is the single most common cause of mental instability. The onset of the condition is rare before the age of 60. Its cause is still relatively unknown, but some research has generated a theory that toxic poisoning from high levels of aluminium could be a contributory factor. Symptoms start with general forgetfulness, progressing to more extreme memory loss, to a state which can eventually lead to complete disorientation and confusion. It is at this stage that full-time care is needed.

MULTIPLE SCLEROSIS

Multiple sclerosis (MS) is a disorder of the central nervous system in which the myelin sheath (the protective covering of the nerve fibres) becomes damaged due to inflammation. As a result the transmission of messages from the brain to the body is disrupted, leading to permanent disability in extreme cases.

The underlying cause of MS is still unknown, but some research suggests that it could be an auto-immune disorder. One link that has been identified between sufferers is an abnormality in the way their bodies treat fats. In particular, the fatty acid, linoleic acid has been found to be lacking in the plasma, red cells and nerve tissues of MS sufferers. It is sometimes genetically inherited and seems to be more common in women. It is not an age-related condition: in fact the onset can be in the 20s or 30s. Symptoms can be varied and include tingling, numbness, weakness on one side of the body, heaviness of a limb and sometimes impaired vision.

WAYS OF HELPING

• Swimming is often recommended as it puts no pressure on the joints.

• Regular physiotherapy treatments . Eat plenty of foods rich in vitamin B. All the B vitamins are essential for a healthy nervous system.

• Take evening primrose oil or sunflower oil which are good sources of linoleic acid.

The Multiple Sclerosis Society (see page 218) offers practical help and counselling.

PARKINSON'S DISEASE

Parkinson's disease is a neurological disorder resulting from degeneration of the nerve cells within the basal ganglia (paired nerve cell clusters in the brain responsible for smooth muscle movement). The underlying cause of the disease is a deficiency of brain dopamine (a neurotransmitter). Clinically this condition can lead to three major symptoms: impairment or slowness of movements; muscle rigidity, leading to almost complete immobility; and tremor of limbs, head or lower jaw. It occurs mainly in elderly people and tends to be more common in men.

The symptoms usually start with slight tremors in the head, arm or leg and may be worse while resting. As the condition progresses stiffness, weakness and a more pronounced trembling, shaking of the head, problems with balance and slurred speech develop. Sometimes the intelligence remains unaffected. As yet there is no cure for disease, but research has been carried out on use of the the broad bean plant *Vicia fava*. It is a natural source of the amino acid *L Dopa* which human brain cells lose the capability to synthesize as they age.

WAYS OF HELPING

The following methods should relieve some of the symptoms:

• Homeopathy.

• Reflexology.

• Acupuncture.

• Massage.

• Relaxation.

Counselling or psychotherapy can also assist sufferers in coming to terms with their condition.

Endocrine

FUNCTION

The endocrine system comprises the following glands, each with responsibility for a different cellular function:

• The pituitary gland.

• The pineal gland.

• The thyroid gland.

• Four parathyroid glands.

• Two adrenal glands.

• The islets of Langerhans in the pancreas.

• Two ovaries in the female and two testes in the male.

The endocrine system serves as a regulator and integrator of cellular functions and organ systems, and consists of endocrine or ductless glands which secrete hormones directly into the bloodstream. All the glands interact with and depend on each other and the hormones they secrete are essential for regulating all the vital functions and metabolic processes necessary for good health.

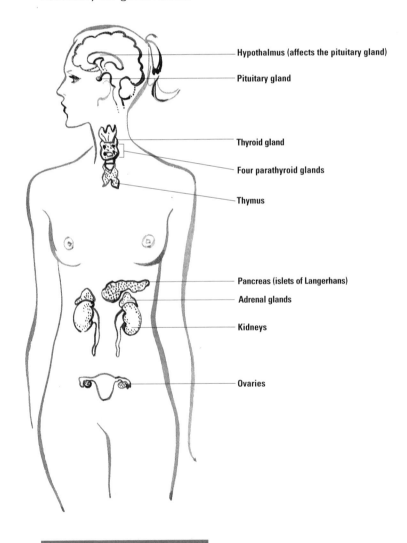

- Hypothalmus (affects the pituitary gland)
- Pituitary gland
- Thyroid gland
- Four parathyroid glands
- Thymus
- Pancreas (islets of Langerhans)
- Adrenal glands
- Kidneys
- Ovaries

THE GLANDS

The pituitary gland Although only the size of a pea, the pituitary is the main endocrine gland. It is responsible for the body's growth and also assists the function of the other glands. The hypothalamus, although not an endocrine gland, has a direct effect on the pituitary. It connects the nervous and endocrine systems and has many important functions, such as regulating the heart and abdominal organs, controlling our emotions, regulating body temperature, controlling appetite and thirst and, most important, governing the secretion of hormones from the pituitary gland.

The pineal gland Another tiny pea-sized gland, the pineal secretes melatonin, a hormone which, scientists are now discovering, could have many long-term benefits. This tiny gland has a direct influence on our behaviour and moods.

The thyroid and parathyroid glands The main function of the thyroid gland is to control metabolism through its secretion of thyroxine. The parathyroid glands, which lie behind the thyroid, ensure adequate concentration of calcium salts in both the blood and bone structure.

The adrenal glands The outer part of the adrenal controls the body's balance of sodium and potassium, water, acid and sex hormones and regulates glucose metabolism. The inner section secretes adrenaline, known as the 'fight or flight' hormone because it controls our reaction to stress or shock.

The pancreas (islets of Langerhans) The endocrine part of the pancreas, which is also an exocrine gland, secretes insulin. This regulates the level of sugar in the blood and its conversion of heat into energy.

The ovaries The ovaries secrete oestrogen and progesterone and are responsible for all the manifestations of femininity and female reproduction.

LOCATION

The glands in the body are located as follows:

- **Pituitary** Suspended from the base of the brain.
- **Pineal** In the fore brain.
- **Thyroid** At the base of the throat.
- **Parathyroids** Behind each of the four corners of the thyroid.
- **Adrenals** On top of each kidney.
- **Islets of Langerhans** In the pancreas.
- **Ovaries** In the lower pelvic region.

Oestrogen & progesterone

The word oestrogen comes from the Latin *oestrus*, meaning the time when female animals are on heat. Doctors first identified this female sex hormone in 1929. Not only is it important for reproduction and fertility, but it controls 300 different functions in the female body, crucial to our health and wellbeing.

Oestrogen is not a single hormone. There are three different types: oestradiol which is produced mainly by the ovaries and is the dominant hormone during pregnancy; and oestrone and oestriol which are produced by the adrenal hormones in the adrenal glands. After the menopause the ovaries still produce oestrogen, but the main source is oestrone, which is converted from fatty tissue. Oestrogen is needed for smooth joint mobility and its decrease after the menopause may account for many women's experience of aching joints and arthritic conditions during and after this time. It is also needed for maintaining healthy skin tone and texture, healthy hair, heart and blood vessels, muscle tone and strength and strong healthy bones, and especially during pregnancy and breastfeeding for assisting the production of the baby's bones. Mucous membranes such as those in the eyes, mouth and vagina rely on oestrogen for moisture. Memory and mood can also be affected by oestrogen levels as they affect certain neurotransmitters which help to control the production of oestrogen. This is thought to be an important contributory factor in PMT, post-natal depression and around the menopause – all times when hormonal imbalance is prevalent. Oestrogen also works in close harmony with other hormones produced by the ovaries: progesterone, the male sex hormone testosterone and small amounts of other male hormones.

Progesterone is a single hormone. In the ovaries it is a precursor of oestrogen, and small amounts are also produced by the adrenal glands. Corticosteroids, which are essential to our body's response to stress, our blood pressure and sugar and electrolyte balance, are also derived from progesterone.

Oestrogen is the primary hormone during the first two weeks of the menstrual cycle, preparing the endometrium for pregnancy, whereas progesterone is the major reproductive hormone during the latter half of the cycle. It is the delicate balance of the two which is so important to a woman's health.

Does oestrogen deficiency really exist?

Although menopause is associated with a decrease in oestrogen levels, Dr Carolyn DeMarco, author of *Take Charge of Your Body* and a physician specializing in women's health issues, says there is no direct proof that lack of oestrogen causes heart disease or any other ailments associated with the menopause. Dr Jerilyn Prior, researcher and Professor of Endocrinology at the University of British Columbia in Vancouver, similarly believes that the relationship between oestrogen deficiency, menopausal symptoms and related diseases is still unclear due to lack of conclusive research.

Oestrogen dominance

Dr John Lee, a retired medical practitioner from California, has spent years researching female problems such as PMT, ovarian cysts, fibroids, breast cancer, endometriosis and menopausal problems. His belief is that in fact many women are suffering from too much oestrogen.

His findings indicate that nutritional deficiencies, stress, taking synthetic oestrogens, and oestrogenic substances in our environment such as pesticides, herbicides and certain plastics, combined with a resulting deficiency of progesterone are very likely contributing factors to oestrogen dominance. Oestrogen mimics, called xeno-oestrogens, are polluting the air, water and soil and have a powerful oestrogenic effect on our bodies. They are fat-soluble, non-biodegradable and highly toxic.

He believes that symptoms exacerbated by oestrogen dominance can be counteracted by increasing the level of natural progesterone, not because progesterone levels in such cases are lower but because they are low in comparison to the elevated oestrogen levels. Natural progesterone is derived from wild or Mexican yam, a plant extract containing diosgenin, the raw material from which synthetic progesterone is made.

SYMPTOMS

The following symptoms may be linked to oestrogen dominance:

- Breast tenderness.
- Decreased sex drive.
- Depression.
- Thinning hair or excessive facial hair.
- Fibrocystic breasts.
- Hypoglycaemia (low blood sugar).
- Increased blood clotting and risk of stroke.
- Infertility and miscarriage,
- Osteoporosis and pre-menopausal bone loss.
- Water retention, bloating and fat gain (especially around the hips, abdomen and thighs).
- Auto-immune disorders such as thyroiditis and lupus.
- PMT.
- Speeding of the ageing process.

HYPOTHYROIDISM

Hypothyroidism (underactive thyroid gland) is one of the more common disorders of the endocrine system. It often goes undiagnosed, but if you suffer with this condition it can affect your body, your emotions – indeed, your whole life. The thyroid controls metabolism, the rate at which normal chemical processes interact within the body and the speed at which the body burns fuel (the food which we eat and the oxygen in the air we breathe). Proper working of every cell, every organ and every process in the body is essential for health and well-being. A healthy metabolism controls the way in which the body reacts to and throws off illness and disease.

Hypothyroidism is far more common in women than in men and can be a slow, progressive process. Women seem to be particularly vulnerable after childbirth, or gynaecological problems perhaps involving hysterectomy. Major injuries, car accidents, operations (especially tonsillectomy in adults), and glandular fever are often the instigators of hypothyroidism. Symptoms such as tiredness, lethargy, weight gain, digestive problems, cold hands and feet, dry skin, thinning hair, heavy periods, puffiness of the face and eyes and lack of sex drive are all so common that the thyroid often goes unsuspected. A simple blood test will confirm the condition.

HYPERTHYROIDISM

Hyperthyroidism (overactive thyroid gland) is not as common as hypothyroidism. Symptoms usually include a rapid heartbeat, irritability, nervousness, weight loss and weakness. Genetics can play a part in all thyroid conditions, as can physical injury and severe mental stress.

GRAVE'S DISEASE

Grave's disease is a specific form of thyroid overactivity which often arises as a result of hyperthyroidism. It is thought to be due to the body producing an 'autoantibody'. The thyroid becomes enlarged and it can sometimes lead to the toxic condition, thyrotoxicosis.

Adrenal syndrome

Low-functioning adrenal glands cause a weakness in the body's ability to respond to stress. The symptoms are a tendency towards low blood pressure, sensitivity to cold, poor circulation, cold hands and feet, continual exhaustion and oversensitivity to allergic or environmental substances.
At such adrenal lows, our body tends to rely on our anti-stress hormones (steroids) and hormones such as cortisone. This has anti-inflammatory properties and delays the proliferative changes in tissue which are the normal response to infections and allergies.

Contributory factors towards adrenal syndrome/insufficiency are similar to those affecting the thyroid and include injury, illness, accident and gynaecological problems (especially hysterectomy or menopause), when the adrenal glands are looked toward for their reserve. The constant stress which many people endure nowadays is, on its own, a frequent cause of adrenal exhaustion. People with a thyroid condition will also often suffer with adrenal problems as the functions of the two types of gland are interlinked.

WAYS OF HELPING
• Reduce your stress levels.
• Increase vitamin C intake which helps to produce cortisone.
• Increase your intake of pantothenic acid (a precursor to cortisone), found in broccoli, watercress, peas, lentils, tomatoes, cabbage, celery, eggs, strawberries, avocado and alfalfa.

Diabetes

Diabetes is due to lack of insulin from the pancreas, needed to regulate blood sugar levels. It can be hereditary, or sometimes a viral infection can trigger off the illness. When there is an insulin deficiency, the body's cell receptors are not properly opened, thereby preventing glucose from entering, and the result is an excess of sugar in the bloodstream which can cause various problems. Diabetics face the risk of stroke, heart disease, kidney disease and impaired vision.

There are two types of diabetes: juvenile diabetes which is often diagnosed during puberty, and adult-onset diabetes, which is more common and can strike women during their late 40s. Symptoms include recurring gum, bladder and skin infections, slow-healing cuts and sometimes a slight tingling in the hands and feet. The symptoms can go unnoticed so it is important to have regular blood sugar level tests.

WAYS OF HELPING
• Avoid becoming overweight.
• Maintain a healthy diet low in sugar and salt and high in fibre as the latter is thought to reduce the body's need for insulin.
• Control stress as it drains the adrenal glands which help to control blood sugar levels.
• Take regular exercise, but with caution, or there could be a risk of hypoglycaemia (low blood sugar).
• Try chromium supplements which have been shown through trials to assist blood sugar levels.

Immune

FUNCTION

The immune system is the body's defence system against attack by bacteria, viruses and even cancer cells. It consists of:

• **The thymus gland located behind the breastbone.**

• **Several types of white blood cells, which produce antibodies and attack viruses.**

• **Bone marrow which manufactures some white blood cells.**

• **The spleen.**

• **Lymph nodes and lymph ducts.**

A healthy immune system is essential for life and the benefits it provides are proof of its power within the body. On a cellular level the work is done through the B cells, T cells and macrophages. B cells, which are made in the bone marrow, produce antibodies against infection. T cells are manufactured in the thymus gland which directs the time and line of attack. Without the correct information from the thymus these T cells could fail to perform the necessary assault on bacteria, viruses and cancer cells. Macrophages are large cells which engulf bacteria and other foreign particles.

AGEING AND THE IMMUNE SYSTEM

The body's immune system is at its prime around the time of puberty, after which the thymus gland begins to shrink, thereby affecting T cell production and functioning. In theory the T cells are left to recognize foreign invaders on their own without the influence of the thymus gland. All in all the disappearance of the thymus and the decline in the cell production and function causes this extremely intricate system to gradually become less proficient. During the ageing process the immune system loses its capacity to distinguish foreign substances and actively begins to destroy its own army. This is known as auto-immunity and is thought to be one of the main underlying procedures of ageing.

LOW-FUNCTIONING IMMUNE SYSTEM

When the immune system is weak, the body becomes vulnerable to illnesses from the common cold, throat infections and thrush to the more serious auto-immune diseases such as arthritis. The best recourse is to prevent infection from starting at all by taking steps to reduce those factors that are thought to be responsible for a low immune system. Other than the unavoidable factor of one's heredity and genetic make-up, the following can all have a detrimental effect:

Stress The adrenal glands have to work overtime during periods of stress and the adrenaline and steroids which are produced consequently suppress the functioning of the immune system cells. We can work to reduce stress levels through relaxation, meditation, yoga and enjoyable hobbies.

Lack of sleep While we sleep the immune system nourishes and strengthens the defence mechanisms in the body. During sleep, when the body is resting, there is less of a struggle to obtain the necessary nutrients. Without enough sleep the immune system will suffer.

Smoking The body has to deal with the foreign substances present in tobacco which affect the condition of the lungs, causing a greater susceptibility to colds and chest problems. Therefore one of the greatest boosts you can give your immune system is to give up smoking.

Poor nutrition Refined and processed foods contain 'empty' nutrients and toxins which the body cannot handle easily. It then has the task of eliminating them. To increase your immunity, vitamins A, C, D and E and the mineral zinc are particularly beneficial (see chapter five for sources).

Lack of exercise Exercise oxygenates the blood, increases circulation, detoxifies the lungs and increases perspiration which helps to rid the body of toxins. Try gentle exercise such as walking or jogging to improve this.

Environmental pollution We encounter pollutants in every area of life, from those in our water such as aluminium, chlorine or lead, in our food in nitrates from chemically fertilized soil, or in the air from carbon monoxide fumes emitted by cars. These are compounded by the increased levels of radiation. The best way to minimize the effects of pollution is to increase your intake of anti-oxidants which combat free radicals and assist prevention of cancer.

BENEFITS

A healthy immune system will benefit the body in the following ways. It will:
• Clear the body of dead cells and toxic chemicals daily.
• Protect against chemical pollutants and radiation.
• Destroy cancer cells as they are formed.
• Determine the speed of an individual's ageing process.
• Neutralize and destroy micro-organisms wherever they attack the body.
• 'Remember' attackers from the past and prepare for defence.
• Develop a wide range of defences against different pathogens (disease-causing agents).

WAYS OF HELPING

• The supplements and vitamins of most benefit are general multi-vitamin/mineral supplement, B-complex vitamins, magnesium and co-enzyme Q10.

• Get plenty of rest and avoid stress.

• Take herbal remedies echinacea and astragalus to boost the immune system and St John's wort to lift the spirits.

• Bach Flower Remedies, such as Heather for depression, Clematis for low vitality, and Crab Apple to cleanse the system.

POSSIBLE SYMPTOMS

• Total physical exhaustion.
• Chronic muscle fatigue and pain.
• Muscle and limb twitches.
• Headaches and ringing in the ears.
• Visual disturbances and sensitivity to light.
• Swollen glands.
• Candidiasis (thrush).
• Frequent need to pass urine.
• Loss of concentration, short-term memory.
• Mood swings and depression.
• Irritable bowel syndrome.
• Fever and localized sweating.
• Food intolerances.
• Disturbed balance.
• Itchy skin rash or a sensation of pins and needles.

MYALGIC ENCEPHALOMYELITIS (ME)

Myalgic encephalomyelitis (ME), also known as 'yuppie flu' and post-viral syndrome, has often been dismissed as 'all in the mind' or at best simply a reaction to high-pressure modern living. Sufferers have had a real struggle convincing the medical profession that their condition even existed.

It is now estimated that 150,000 people are affected in the UK and not only does the World Health Organization classify it as a disease of the nervous system but the Department of Health now officially recognizes it as a 'debilitating and distressing condition'. ME can hold a person in its grip for years and can affect one's personality, lifestyle and relationships.

According to Dr Charles Shepherd, medical advisor to the ME Association, the cause of ME is still unclear, but in 75 per cent of cases the trigger seems to be some kind of viral illness such as tonsillitis, glandular fever or chickenpox. He is also investigating links between ME and vaccinations, in particular that for hepatitis B, and feels that people exposed to certain pesticides such as those found in pet flea sprays are vulnerable to the disease. A number of studies of ME sufferers also show abnormalities in the hypothalamus (the body's thermostat) and the attached pituitary gland, which would interfere with normal functioning of the brain and give rise to some of the symptoms associated with the disease. Other viruses, such as entero types, which enter the body and multiply in the bowels, may be a trigger for certain people. Medical researchers have found a disturbed immune system and changes in the composition of muscle cells in some ME sufferers. Another factor often shared by these sufferers is physical or emotional stress.

ME is often misdiagnosed as irritable bowel syndrome from the similarity of the symptoms. Food intolerance is frequently a contributory factor to ME and many sufferers find that excluding suspect foods such as wheat and dairy products brings about an improvement. It is important to test for food intolerances – there are various methods (see page 204) – and to acquire professional nutritional advice. A wholefood diet based on unprocessed foods will probably be suggested.

There is no conventional treatment for ME, but there are various ways of helping towards recovery, albeit slowly – it can take a long time to rebuild the immune system. Many complementary therapies are beneficial as the therapists will address the problem from a holistic viewpoint, approaching the cause of the illness according to the physiological and emotional needs of the individual patient. Acupuncture, aromatherapy, yoga, homeopathy, reflexology and naturopathy are often used as ways to relieve the stress, tiredness and depression associated with the disease. Contact The ME Association about self-help groups (see page 218).

COLDS AND FLU

Colds are caused by virus infections and are extremely contagious. Babies, young children, the elderly and those who are already ill are particularly at risk as their immune systems are less resistant, and they should try and avoid people who are infected. It is easy to spread a cold, especially in enclosed places, simply through breathing, sneezing and coughing as the virus lies in the mucus in the nasal and throat areas and tiny disease-filled droplets are propelled into the air. Symptoms are usually a headache, sore throat, cough, sneezing, reduced appetite and a general feeling of being 'run down'. Some colds last only a few days, others may linger for two to three weeks. A cold may also be accompanied by other complaints such as bronchitis, sinus infection and middle ear infection.

Influenza, more commonly called flu, is a viral infection of the respiratory tract. Like colds it is spread by coughing, sneezing and breathing the virus-infected droplets of mucus into the air. The symptoms are similar to those of the common cold, but chill, fever and muscular aches are usually present as well. It is important for the elderly or anyone who suffers with heart or lung disease to seek prompt medical attention as soon as any symptoms develop. Anti-flu vaccines are available containing strains of different types of the virus but any immunity provided needs to be repeated each year. It is advisable to keep the immune system as healthy and protective as possible.

WAYS OF HELPING

• Keep the head warm – about 80 per cent of the body's heat can be lost through the head.

• Eat garlic or take supplements.

• Drink plenty of fluids, preferably water or herbal tea.

• Avoid mucus-forming foods such as milk and dairy products.

• Eat plenty of raw or steamed vegetables and fruit.

• Take 1g of vitamin C every hour at the first sign of a cold. If diarrhoea develops, slightly reduce the dose.

• Steam inhalations with a few drops of eucalyptus, peppermint oil and camphor help clear the sinuses. Eucalyptus and camphor added to a cream or oil base make a chest rub.

• Half teaspoon hot lemon juice and 1 teaspoon honey in a cup of hot water makes a soothing drink.

• Try massaging some of the Shiatsu facial points (see page 135) to relieve headaches and painful sinuses.

WAYS OF HELPING

• Many of the holistic therapies have benefited HIV and AIDS sufferers. These include autogenic training, body stress release, naturopathy, acupuncture, massage, aromatherapy, reflexology and herbal medicine (see chapter two).

• Some of the Bach Flower Remedies (see chapters two and three) are also very helpful for the emotional feelings associated with this condition, such as guilt, fear of getting ill, fear of death and feelings of resentment.

• High doses of vitamin C can boost the immune system.

• The herbs echinacea and astragalus are also known to benefit the immune system. A diet rich in anti-oxidant foods is beneficial, or a dietary supplement containing vitamins A, C, E beta-carotene and selenium.

• Avoid fungi, yeast and sugar if you suffer from thrush.

• Relieve stress using yoga and meditation.

The national AIDS Helpline offers free confidential information, advice and support 24 hours a day, seven days a week (see page 218).

HIV AND AIDS

AIDS (acquired immune deficiency syndrome) is caused by a virus – namely HIV (human immuno-deficiency virus) – against which the body has no defence. This is because the virus attacks the T cells which, in a normal healthy person, help the body to fight off infection. As yet there is no cure for AIDS.

HIV is transmitted via the bodily fluids, such as blood or semen, of an infected person usually as a result of sexual intercourse, oral sex, injection with a contaminated hypodermic needle, passing of the infection from mother to foetus, or transfusion with contaminated blood or blood products (though donated blood is thoroughly screened). On occasions it can be passed through artificial-insemination-by-donor semen, although tests are now carried out to prevent this.

HIV can cause devastating damage to the immune system and it is the severity of this damage together with the functioning of the individual's immune system which determine the course of the disease. Actual symptoms of full-blown AIDS such as lung infections, disorders of the nervous and digestive systems and certain cancers (such as cervical cancer in women and Kaposi's sarcoma in men) may not occur for about eight to ten years, but symptoms develop in three out of every ten people with HIV. Others remain carriers of the virus and sometimes stay reasonably well: no one is exactly sure of the reason for this, but maintaining a healthy immune system and a positive mental attitude and living as healthy and stress-free a lifestyle as possible will help.

Early symptoms of HIV are usually lymph gland enlargement in the neck, groin or armpits, marked weight loss, diarrhoea, oral thrush, skin problems such as dermatitis, fever and muscle pain. Later on severe symptoms can develop such as shingles, herpes simplex, tuberculosis and bowel disorders.

To guard against contracting AIDS it is advisable to practise safe sex and avoid the use of shared needles. If there is any doubt about whether you have contracted the virus, and if you are thinking about becoming pregnant, it is wise to obtain counselling with a view to undergoing a blood test.

CANCER

Cancer is the development of abnormal cells in a particular area of the body due to the confusion of normal cell division. Every six months the body's cells are replaced; normally reproducing by dividing into two. At the centre of each cell lie the controls for genetic coding which determine the development and behaviour of the cells. In some cases abnormal cells develop which multiply uncontrollably because of a defect in their coding. When this happens, cancer develops. The most prevalent forms of the condition are lung cancer (more common in men); prostate in men; breast and cervical cancer in women; and skin cancer and bowel cancer, affecting either sex. Heredity is a risk factor in certain cancers. Fair-skinned, light-haired people are more likely to develop skin cancer. Bowel problems such as ulcerative colitis could prove a risk in developing bowel cancer. Environmental factors have been shown to play a part: for example, passive smoking and over-exposure to sunlight and certain chemicals can cause cancer.

Some cancers can take years to develop, which is why it is so important to improve diet and lifestyle now as a prevention. If cancer has been diagnosed, it should not be thought of as automatically terminal. Increasing life force through improving the body's defence system can prevent or help the illness.

The power of positive thinking

Positive thinking can be a powerful tool whether you have to deal with cancer on your own behalf or as a carer for someone else. Penny Brohn, co-founder of the Bristol Cancer Help Centre, firmly believes in the power of hope. Whatever form it takes, it can lead to action by helping you to face up to the problem and then deal with it. The Centre runs courses for both cancer patients and their carers (see page 218).

Dr Ian Gowler successfully fought his own cancer and now runs his own support centre in Australia with his wife. He believes in combating cancer with a fighting spirit and the courage to realize your dreams. To this end he has identified five stages of hope experienced by cancer patients.

WAYS OF HELPING

• Give up smoking.
• Reduce your alcohol intake.
• Increase dietary fibre to maintain a healthy colon.
• Include in your diet plenty of anti-oxidant foods such as fresh fruit, vegetables, oily fish, nuts and seeds. Anthocyanidins, such as grapeseed and bilberry extract, are very powerful anti-oxidants, as is Quercitin.
• Reduce fat intake.
• Be careful not to char food too much when barbecuing.
• Avoid prolonged exposure to the sun.
• Check your family medical history for any genetic roots to cancer.
• Have regular cervical smears and mammograms and check your breasts for lumps (see page 57).

FIVE STAGES OF HOPE

• The belief that desirable things can be obtained to bring you out of despair.
• Hope for survival: focusing on avoiding death rather than living well.
• Hope for a better future: life will be fulfilling again so try to help yourself.
• Hope for spiritual realization: a spiritual path will lead to a state of completion.
• Hope for fulfilment in the present – the realization that this very moment is sufficient and complete.

Lymphatic

FUNCTION

The lymphatic system is a drainage system for the circulation, serves a function in immunity and also plays a part in the absorption of fats from the intestines.

Occasionally you may notice tender swellings in the neck, groin or underarm areas. This is due to inflammation of the lymph nodes. Within the lymphatic system, waste and other substances from the cells are carried to the heart through lymph vessels which contain a clear body fluid called lymph. On the way to the heart there are little reservoirs known as lymph nodes and these act as filters to prevent infection from spreading into the bloodstream by neutralizing or destroying bacteria. In their fight against harmful bacteria white blood cells can accumulate in these lymph nodes causing inflammation.

The largest lymph nodes are in the neck, armpits, elbows, groin and backs of knees and the main lymphatic ducts are in the chest. The lymph ducts drain into the veins, completing the journey to the heart and back into the bloodstream.

WAYS OF HELPING

To reduce the chances of developing cellulite:

• **Eat more lean meat, fish and vegetables and fewer dairy products, sugary and refined foods.**
• **Avoid coffee. Caffeine puts stress on the kidneys and adrenal glands.**
• **Give up smoking.**
• **Reduce your alcohol consumption.**
• **Increase the amount of regular aerobic exercise you take.**
• **Drink plenty of water.**
• **Body brushing can help (see page 196).**
• **Massage using essential oils juniper, cypress, lemon, rosemary or black pepper. Also readily available are anti-cellulite massage blends.**

CELLULITE

Cellulite is the main problem associated with a sluggish lymphatic system. It occurs through a combination of fluid retention and hardened collagen and elastin fibres in the skin, which causes fat to be 'squeezed' into nodules, producing the 'orange peel' effect. It mainly affects the thighs, buttocks and upper arms and usually feels cold to the touch due to poor circulation. Cellulite is a definite indication of a toxic build-up within the body which it is unable to handle so it uses these areas as 'dumping grounds'. In order to detoxify we must work at keeping the liver and kidneys free to eliminate the toxins.

Cellulite is also linked to the hormonal system and the presence of oestrogen, which is why some contraceptive pills actually encourage it. Puberty, pregnancy and menopause are likely times to develop this condition, but stress can also trigger off cellulite since it can affect the lymphatic circulation causing lymphatic fluid and waste. Sometimes there can be a hereditary tendency to develop cellulite, but not surprisingly given the hormonal influence, men are rarely affected.

THE LYMPH NODES

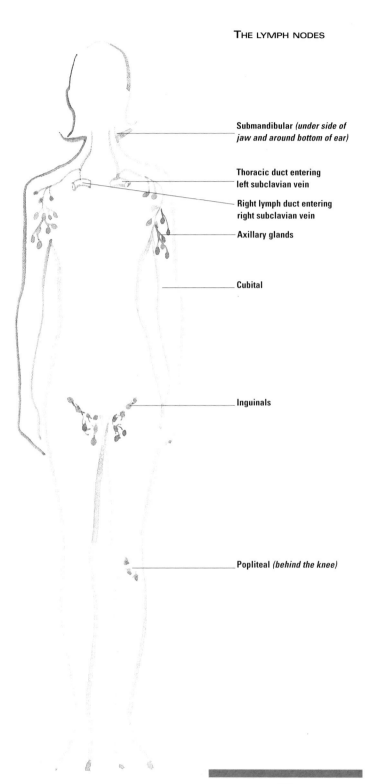

Submandibular *(under side of jaw and around bottom of ear)*

Thoracic duct entering left subclavian vein

Right lymph duct entering right subclavian vein

Axillary glands

Cubital

Inguinals

Popliteal *(behind the knee)*

HELPING YOUR LYMPHATIC SYSTEM

Unlike the vascular system the lymphatic system has no pumping action to assist it, but the following keep it in good order:

• Exercise which increases the flow of lymph around the body.

• Correct breathing.

• Relaxation, meditation, yoga and massage which all help to detoxify and cleanse the lymphatics.

• The diaphragm itself which acts as a pump to assist the system.

Digestive

FUNCTION

The function of the digestive system is to convert the food we consume into substances suitable for absorption and use by the body. The digestive tract, if laid out, would be the length of a football pitch. It begins at the mouth, passes though the pharynx, oesophagus (gullet), stomach, small and large intestines and finally the rectum and anus. Associated with it are the accessory organs such as: the tongue, the teeth, the salivary glands and the liver and pancreas.

Our health and energy levels are determined by the foods we ingest. Digestion starts with the senses, when the smell of good food activates chemical reactions which prepare us for its digestion and assimilation. The digestive tract has not changed in the last million years but our diet has altered dramatically in the last hundred, giving rise to numerous problems.

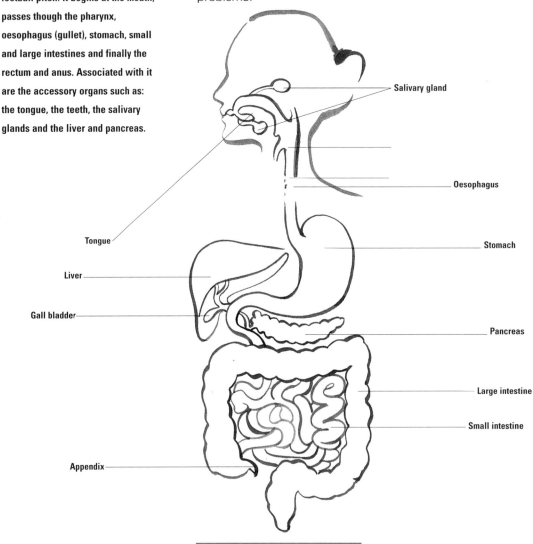

- Salivary gland
- Oesophagus
- Tongue
- Liver
- Stomach
- Gall bladder
- Pancreas
- Large intestine
- Small intestine
- Appendix

Our digestive system was designed for nature's diet and not all the refined and processed foods available today which lack the necessary vitamins, minerals and fibre. Unfortunately many modern meals are prepared and eaten away from home, so we are sometimes completely unaware of all the contents of our food, which may not be beneficial. However, the lining of the digestive tract replaces itself every four days therefore giving us tremendous scope for healing. Another important aspect of healthy digestion is the correct balance of acid and alkalinity within the digestive tract. The mouth and oesophagus are alkaline, the stomach is acid, the duodenum and small intestine are alkaline, and the colon or large intestine are acid. For digestion to be satisfactorily completed, it is important that each section maintains its balance.

Bad digestion is at the root of most illnesses as it has a profound effect on the functioning of the other systems of the body. The saying 'you are what you eat' is only half the story: more important is 'you are what you absorb'.

There are numerous digestive disorders. Common ones include: constipation, indigestion, irritable bowel syndrome, gallstones, ulcers and hiatus hernia.

CONSTIPATION

Difficulty or infrequency in having bowel movements is known as constipation. Unfortunately it has become an increasingly common problem in the western world, mainly as a result of a diet lacking in fibre which is needed to stimulate intestinal action. In western society a lot of people also eat far more food than they really need, so overloading the system.

Although constipation is not a disease in itself, there are a number of symptoms associated with it, such as headaches, abdominal pain, bloating, flatulence, lower back pain, skin problems and general lethargy. It is fairly common during pregnancy due to the extra pressure on the colon, and in some elderly people weakness of the abdominal muscles lowers the peristaltic action and pressure when attempting a bowel movement. People with a low-functioning thyroid gland can

HELPING YOUR DIGESTION

To keep your digestion in good working order and to avoid unnecessary problems, the following elementary methods will help:

• Take care to eat a well balanced nutritious diet through awareness of the value of different foods (see chapter five).

• Chew as you eat. This produces the digestive juices which breakdown the food before it enters the stomach.

• Avoid stress as it diverts adrenaline from the digestive tract and into the muscles, leaving the digestive system functioning less effectively.

WAYS OF HELPING

• Chew food thoroughly.

• Linseeds, sprinkled over cereals or soups or swallowed with water will have a laxative effect.

• Psyllium husks are a soluble fibre which will increase bowel activity. Drink with plenty of water.

• Fructo-oligo saccharides from chicory root, garlic, artichokes and onions prepare the intestines for healthy bacterial growth and help to maintain bowel regularity.

• Epsom salts have a gentle laxative effect. The salts contain magnesium sulphate which assists muscle relaxation and combines well with a high-fibre diet. Pre-menstrual constipation may be caused by lower magnesium levels at this time.

• Exercise motivates digestion and strengthens stomach and back muscles.

• A neck and back massage will stimulate the the vagus nerve which is linked to the digestive system. The lumber spinal nerves feed the internal organs within the pelvic girdle.

suffer constipation as colonic contractions become slower. The adrenal glands, working alongside the thyroid, and controlling intestinal muscle tone and action can also be affected. Long-term use of laxatives can irritate and weaken the tone of the bowel, aggravating the problem. Medications, such as anti-depressants and strong pain killers, can cause constipation. Dehydration or lack of water is another common cause of constipation. The human body is about 60-70 per cent water, which is being used up or lost all the time in urine formation, perspiration and exhalation and constantly needs replacing. We need to drink at least 2 litres/3½ pints of water daily (bottled preferably and not carbonated) and eat a lot of fruits and vegetables which have a high natural water content.

Stress is another common, though not always recognized cause of constipation. Anger, resentment and fear are often held in the pelvic area, resulting in a number of problems. Correct functioning of the colon is vital for good health. It is thought that 80 per cent of all diseased states are the result of an unhealthy colon, putting a strain on other eliminative organs such as the kidneys, lungs and skin. Chronic constipation can lead to further complications such as haemorrhoids, colitis, diverticulitis and even bowel cancer.

Although there are immediate measures you can take to relieve acute constipation, ideally you should aim to prevent it happening again. The easiest way to do this is to reassess your diet. Many people who suffer from constipation are not including enough fibre in their diet. Make sure you eat plenty of fresh fruit and vegetables – pears and raspberries are especially effective. You should also drink as much water as possible – at least 2-3 litres/3½–5 pints daily. Within your diet, try to avoid gluten which is found in meat, cheese, eggs, refined grains and wheat because it has a constipating effect. Wheat bran should also be avoided as it is rather indigestible and may cause a production of gas in the colon from fermentation by bacteria. Wheat bran also prevents the absorption of calcium, magnesium, iron, zinc, copper and other nutrients due to its phytic acid content. It is better to eat oat bran instead.

INDIGESTION

Indigestion is usually caused by eating too much too quickly, or it may be due to incorrect acid balance in the stomach. It is important to produce enough hydrochloric acid to digest protein. The symptoms are usually heartburn, belching, acid regurgitation and nausea. Many of the symptoms can be reduced by simple regulation of when and how you eat. Avoid eating late at night, and learn to eat slowly, chewing properly and to relax during mealtimes. Rich, high fat foods, alcohol, caffeine and carbonated drinks can all contribute to indigestion. Aspririn, although an unlikely culprit, can also exacerbate the problem. Avoid it especially where there is a history of gastric troubles as it can cause internal bleeding.

WAYS OF HELPING

• Drink peppermint, fennel or camomile tea to calm the digestive tract.

• Slippery elm powder or capsules can soothe tissues and mucous membranes of the digestive tract.

• Take supplements of digestive enzymes such as lipase, protease and amylase.

• Take betaine hydrochloride to help break down food in the gut.

• Take bromelain and papain to help digest starches.

IRRITABLE BOWEL SYNDROME

Irritable bowel syndrome (IBS), also known as spastic colon, is a very common problem often associated with other bowel conditions. Twice as common in women than in men, it can sometimes develop after hysterectomy or ovarian surgery. In cases of ulcerative colitis (inflammation of the colon) IBS symptoms can occur. Diverticulosis (a ballooning of the walls of the colon), which is more common in elderly people and results from weakness in the bowel musculature, may also bring about IBS-related symptoms.

The cause of IBS is not fully understood. There are many possibilities such as food intolerance, involuntary muscle weakness in the large intestine, the inability to digest food properly, fermentation in the intestines and stress and anxiety. It cannot always be cured as such, but it can be managed. The symptoms are usually constipation, diarrhoea or both intermittently. Constipation alone can also often develop into IBS. Abdominal pain, abdominal bloating, excessive wind, mucus in the stools, lower back ache, lack of energy and a feeling of incomplete evacuation are common. It is not necessary for sufferers to endure such exhausting symptoms for an extended period of time. If the measures suggested opposite still bring little relief, do consult a doctor.

WAYS OF HELPING

• For diarrhoea avoid spicy foods, and reduce your intake of citrus fruit.

• For wind and bloating avoid sugar, wheat, refined carbohydrates, pulses (dried beans) and broccoli or cabbage.

• Drink peppermint tea or take peppermint oil capsules to relax spasms.

• Aloe vera has been known to relieve IBS symptoms.

• Pantothenic acid aids functioning of the gastro-intestinal tract.

• Fructo oligosaccharides promote probiotic activity and a healthy bowel.

• Pro-biotics like acidophilus bifidus help regulate intestinal bacteria.

• Massage the abdomen in a clockwise direction with essential oils of camomile, rosemary or lavender in a base oil.

• Avoid caffene based drinks.

• Avoid stress.

WAYS OF HELPING

• **Avoid becoming overweight.**

• **Limit your sugar intake.**

• **Reduce your saturated fat intake by cutting down on red meat and dairy products.**

• **Include plenty of fibre in your diet in the form of fresh fruit, vegetables and oat bran.**

• **Psyllium husks and pectin help increase fibre intake.**

• **Lecithin granules to increase cholesterol solubility can be beneficial.**

• **Vitamin C and phosphatidyl choline can lower cholesterol.**

• **Milk thistle herb can help in cleansing the liver and stimulating bile secretion.**

GALLSTONES

The gallbladder stores a substance produced by the liver called bile, which is our own internal 'washing-up liquid' for fats. It emulsifies them into droplets which can then be absorbed into the lymphatic system.

Gallstones develop when there is an imbalance in the chemical composition of the bile. They are insoluble deposits usually formed from excess cholesterol or calcium which combines with bile and crystallize out of solution to form stones. The solubility of bile is dependant on the correct balance being maintained in the gallbladder between cholesterol, bile acids, phosphatidyl choline and water. Cholesterol is precipitated and stones form when there is an increase in cholesterol or a decrease in bile acids, lecithin or water.

Twice as common in women as in men, gallstones affect 10 per cent of the population over 40, although only 20 per cent of cases experience symptoms or complications. Overweight women are particularly prone to this condition. Gallstones are largely attributed to the western diet of low fibre, highly refined foods.

The symptoms are indigestion, intolerance of fatty foods, flatulence, sometimes jaundice, and intense pain in the upper right side of the abdomen which is usually due to a stone becoming lodged in the bile duct. Stones that do not cause symptoms can be left alone and there are continuing developments in ways of disintegrating stones and avoiding surgical removal of the gallbladder.

STOMACH AND DUODENAL ULCERS

Ulcers do not suddenly happen overnight, but are usually the outcome of years of bad diet and/or stress. There are generally early-warning signs in the form of digestive upsets which, if ignored, may lead to ulcers many years later. In the case of stomach (gastric or peptic) ulcers there is often pain immediately after eating, whereas in the case of duodenal ulcers the pain usually arises some time later.

Stomach ulcers tend to occur more in early life, whereas

duodenal ulcers are more common in middle age. Lack of mucosal protection (generally provided as a coating by the top layer of cells in the intestinal tract) is a predominant cause of stomach ulcers, whereas duodenal ulcers are more likely to occur as a result of excess acidity.

Sometimes ulcers are completely 'silent', with no apparent symptoms, but indigestion, heartburn, frequent burping, a burning feeling in the stomach and pain in the upper abdomen are common symptoms. In severe cases of stomach ulcer intense pain in the stomach, vomiting and sometimes a haemorrhage may be experienced. In the case of a duodenal ulcer the pain is felt more in the right side of the abdomen.

Stomach ulcers can be caused by incompatible food combinations, rushed meals, lack of chewing, overuse of laxatives, too much sugar, starch and stress. Stress, anxiety and worry are all emotions which interfere with normal digestive processes. During stressful times the production of gastric juices in the stomach increases and, if there is already a weakening in the stomach lining, these excess juices can cause irritation and ulceration.

WAYS OF HELPING
- Avoid high acid-forming foods such as sugar, red meat, shellfish, pasta and dairy produce.
- Avoid caffeine and alcohol.
- Avoid anti-inflammatory drugs as they can irritate the stomach lining.
- Take slippery elm food as it coats the mucosal lining of the stomach.
- Drink liquorice and cabbage juice.
- Take anti-oxidants (vitamins A, C and E, beta-carotene and selenium).

HIATUS HERNIA

Hiatus hernia occurs when part of the stomach protrudes through the diaphragm where the oesophagus (gullet) passes through the abdominal cavity. This condition seems to be quite common around from the age of 50 upwards. There are often no particular symptoms other than indigestion or heartburn due to excess acid from the stomach flowing into the oesophagus. Diagnosing a hiatus hernia is usually carried out through a barium x-ray examination with the patient lying on tilted bed head down.

Hiatus hernia is more prevalent in overweight people and any pressure on the stomach can worsen the condition. Avoid wearing tight-fitting clothes, lying down after a meal and bending over when the stomach is full. Equally in order to give your digestion the most encouragement at this time, it is a good idea to sleep with the head of the bed raised.

WAYS OF HELPING
- Eat small regular meals.
- Eat your last meal of the day early in the evening.
- Give up smoking and alcohol.
- Avoid foods which cause excessive stomach acid activity, such as tea, coffee, citrus fruits and tomatoes.
- Lose weight if necessary.

Urinary

FUNCTION

The main function of the urinary system is to process, filter and excrete urine. It consists of:

• Two kidneys.

• The renal arteries.

• Two ureters.

• The bladder.

• The urethra.

Much of the active effectiveness of our urinary system is controlled by the workings of the kidneys. These are situated just above the waistline at the back of the abdominal cavity on either side of the spine. They have many functions including: maintaining blood pressure; regulating the body's water content; separating certain waste substances from the blood; producing urine; regulating the body's acid balance; eliminating waste products; and producing hormones. The efficiency of the kidneys gradually diminishes with age as there is a reduction in the number of operational nephrons (filtering funnels). Diabetes also has a damaging effect on the kidneys through excess glucose in the blood which affects the nephrons. Any kidney problems can cause high blood pressure and vice versa – high blood pressure can cause kidney problems.

The most common conditions which can arise within the urinary system are described below. As a general rule they will all be exacerbated by too much animal protein or citrus fruits.

WAYS OF HELPING

• Reduce salt to avoid water retention.

• Drink plenty of water to flush out the bladder and eliminate toxins. Avoid tea and coffee which are irritants.

• Drink barley water or cranberry juice diluted with water.

• Vitamin C, zinc and echinacea and garlic can all help fight infection.

CYSTITIS

Cystitis is inflammation of the inner lining of the bladder and is usually caused by an infection. Unfortunately a woman's 'plumbing system' is rather badly designed compared to that of a man. The distance between the urethra and the bladder is very short in women, which is why they are far more prone to infections than men.

The main symptoms of cystitis are a frequent urge to pass urine often accompanied by pain or a burning sensation.

WAYS OF HELPING

• Drink plenty of water.

• Avoid stimulants like tea and coffee.

• Improve immune system with plenty of Vitamin C and echinacea.

NEPHRITIS

Nephritis is inflammation of one or both kidneys, which can be caused by infection. Antibodies produced by the body can invade the tissue of the kidney. Symptoms include red or cloudy urine, water retention, high blood pressure, backache and headache. It is best to seek medical help if symptoms persist.

KIDNEY STONES

Kidney stones are fairly common and may remain silently in the kidney without any symptoms. Sugar, salt and caffeine will all have a negative effect, but the formation of kidney stones is usually associated with a build up of calcium and unprocessed substances such as dietary fat bonding with it. It is when the stones start to move that the pain, known as renal colic, begins. Symptoms are usually severe lower back pain, painful urination and sometimes blood in the urine.

WAYS OF HELPING
- Drink plenty of water.
- Take vitamin C (especially calcium ascorbate, magnesium ascorbate or ester C) and vitamin B6 which breaks down oxalic acid, a cause of calcium oxalic stones.
- Take potassium to reduce sodium and to balance acid and alkaline levels.

GOUT

Gout is caused by an excess of uric acid in the blood and deposits of uric acid crystals in one or more joints. These crystals can bring on severe pain, making the joint inflamed. Gout often leads to attacks of arthritis. Symptoms are redness, swelling and severe pain, often in the big toe. To reduce the inflammation include in the diet fish oil, vitamin E and bromelain (taken between meals). Gout can also affect other joints, such as the knee, wrist, ankle and the small joints of the hand.

WAYS OF HELPING
- Drink plenty of water to prevent the build-up of crystals in the kidney.
- Cut out alcohol as it increases uric acid build-up.
- Reduce your animal protein intake.
- Celery seeds help clear toxins from the system which affect the buildup of uric acid crystals in the joints.

INCONTINENCE

There are two main types of incontinence – stress incontinence and urge incontinence. Stress incontinence usually happens when coughing or sneezing or during physical exertion and is more common in women. Urge incontinence is usually experienced when there is a sudden and desperate urge to urinate and it feels impossible to 'hold on'. A third type, known as reflex incontinence, can occur as a result of spinal cord injury which prevents the brain from transmitting the message to the bladder that urination should begin. The effect is similar to an irritable bladder when an urge to urinate is persistent but the bladder, contracts involuntarily. People with conditions such as multiple sclerosis, Parkinson's disease or Alzheimer's disease can also experience severe incontinence due to neurological disturbances. Some women may experience a degree of incontincence after childbirth, as the pelvic floor muscles which control urinating have become stretched or weakened.

WAYS OF HELPING
To rebuild and strengthen the pelvic floor muscles if they have become stretched or weakened, try these exercises:
a) While relaxing the stomach and buttocks, hold the vaginal muscles tight then relax. Repeat the exercise a few times each day gradually increasing the 'holding' time.
b) Try starting and stopping the flow of urine for a few seconds while on the toilet and then relax. Repeat daily.
- Cranberry juice alkalizes the system.
- Do not feel embarrassed to discuss this problem with your doctor as it is more common than you think.

Cardiovascular

FUNCTION

The cardiovascular system is vital to the way the body works. It consists of:
- **Blood vessels that carry oxygen, fuel/glucose, amino acids, vitamins and minerals to every cell in the body.**
- **The heart whose main function is to pump oxygenated blood around the body and collect and send the deoxygenated blood back to the lungs for reoxygenating.**

At the centre of this system lies the heart. The heart is divided into four chambers, the right and left atria in the upper part and the right and left ventricles in the lower. It also includes various arteries and veins which carry blood to and from the lungs. The main vessel, the aorta, carries blood all round the body. The blood carrying oxygen, nutrients and anti-bodies, picks up waste products which are filtered by the liver and kidneys.

In the western world heart disease kills more people than any other illness. Although it takes years to develop it can occur at any stage of life. Age brings a general decline in the heart's pumping action and life-threatening obstructions can develop.

HELPING YOUR HEART
- **Reduce intake of saturated fat.**
- **Increase the sources of essential fats in your diet with fresh unsalted nuts, seeds and their unprocessed oils and oily fish such as sardines and mackerel.**
- **Reduce salt intake.**
- **Give up smoking.**
- **Exercise regularly.**
- **Control your stress levels.**
- **Keep your weight under control.**
- **Reduce use of sugar and coffee.**
- **Increase intake of anti-oxidants by eating more fresh fruit and vegetables or taking a supplement containing vitamins A, C and E, beta-carotene and selenium (see chapter five). Vitamin E also protects against cholesterol formation and vitamin C prevents oxidization of cholesterol.**

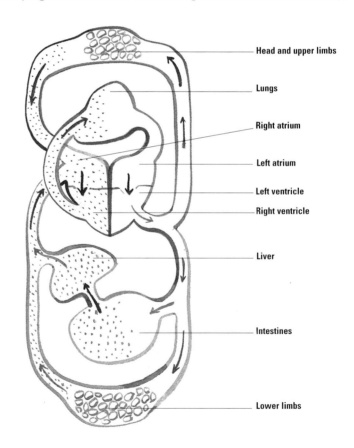

- Head and upper limbs
- Lungs
- Right atrium
- Left atrium
- Left ventricle
- Right ventricle
- Liver
- Intestines
- Lower limbs

ANGINA

Angina is a heart disease caused by narrowing of the coronary arteries, usually due to a build-up of cholesterol and a shortage of blood and oxygen to the heart. In healthy people the flow of blood to the heart keeps pace with demand, but if the demand for oxygen is greater than the supply, the heart is unable to work efficiently. The symptoms of angina range from a tightness in the chest to severe pain which can also be felt in the neck and arms. Angina often occurs when the heart is under pressure such as during stress or physical exertion. Although the symptoms are only temporary, they should be viewed as a warning sign as angina can sometimes lead to further complications, such as a heart attack.

WAYS OF HELPING

The health of the heart muscle can be improved by taking supplements of the following:
- L-carnitine (the amino acid).
- Magnesium.
- Co-enzyme Q10.
- Vitamin E.

CHOLESTEROL

Cholesterol is a substance produced mainly in the liver and it assists the digestion of fats. It also helps to build some of our hormones and to produce vitamin D. For these reasons a certain amount of the right kind of cholesterol is necessary and it is the type of fat we eat which determines this. Consumption of the wrong type of fat can lead to a high build-up of cholesterol in the blood.

Cholesterol travels around the body via the bloodstream, carrying digested fats to the cells. It needs to be packed together with soluble substances called lipoproteins because the blood consists mainly of water, which does not mix with fat. There are two types of lipoprotein: low-density lipoproteins (LDLs) and high-density lipoproteins (HDLs). LDLs pose a health risk as they supply cholesterol to the body tissues and are responsible for its deposit on the artery walls. HDLs remove any 'stuck' cholesterol and transport it back to the liver for disposal or recycling.

It is important to look at the types of fat you eat as well as the amount if you want to lower your cholesterol level. Saturated fats, found in high-fat dairy products, fatty meat and hard margarines made from hydrogenated oils, raise the cholesterol in the blood with LDLs. Monounsaturated and

WAYS OF HELPING

The following methods will help lower your risk of cholesterol build-up.
- Drink skimmed instead of full-fat milk.
- Eat fewer cakes, biscuits, chocolates and crisps.
- Eat lean meat.
- Change to low-fat cheese.
- Avoid deep-fried foods. Instead try microwaving, steaming, boiling and grilling which are much healthier.
- Increase your fibre intake as it helps to lower cholesterol.

polyunsaturated fats, found in foods such as olive oil, actually help the body to produce the more beneficial HDLs.

Cholesterol deposits on the interior walls of the coronary arteries impede blood supply to the heart. Build-up can start at any age, so if you are at all worried, have a cholesterol test. The British Heart Foundation warns against self-tests and mobile cholesterol testing. The only way to diagnose high cholesterol accurately is to have a simple blood text taken by your doctor.

VARICOSE VEINS

WAYS OF HELPING
- Exercise regularly.
- Relax with the feet up.
- Avoid sitting cross-legged.
- Avoid obesity.
- Massage around the affected area, not over it, with a blend of juniper, rosemary and cypress essential oils.
- Silica, vitamins C and E strengthen veins.
- Rutin improves elasticity of veins.
- Avoid tight, restricting clothing.

Varicose veins are abnormally swollen veins, most commonly in the legs. Leg veins contain valves to prevent the blood flowing to the heart and from draining back down the legs through gravity. If these valves malfunction there is a back flow. The veins then swell, and the blood degenerates within them. Women of all ages are prone to varicose veins, particularly during pregnancy, from pressure on the pelvic veins, and during menopause as a result of hormonal changes. People who stand for long periods are also susceptible, and obesity will also encourage them.

If a varicose vein becomes inflamed and the blood clots, the condition is known as phlebitis. Blood clots in the deeper veins (thrombosis) are sometimes linked to variscosities.

HIGH BLOOD PRESSURE

WAYS OF HELPING
- Have regular blood pressure checks.
- Exercise regularly for a healthy heart.
- Give up smoking.
- Reduce your alcohol intake.
- Eat a balanced diet.
- Eat less salt.
- Keep to your ideal weight as excess weight can put a strain on the heart.
- Reduce stress levels by relaxation (see chapter two).

Our blood pressure is constantly changing depending on our activity and circumstances. For instance, it goes down while we are sleeping and it elevates during exercise or when we are stressed, angry or frightened. Without pressure, blood would be unable to flow. However, in some people blood pressure becomes raised above a safe level and it then increases their risk of developing heart disease or stroke.

High blood pressure, (hypertension), has many causes such as a build-up of cholesterol (a type of fat) in the blood, hardening of the arteries, excess smoking, or alcohol, and, of course, stress.

ATHEROSCLEROSIS

Atherosclerosis is narrowing of the arteries caused by plaques on their inner linings and is the most common type of arteriosclerosis (a group of disorders which result in thickening of and loss of elasticity in the artery walls). Atheroma or fatty deposits become stuck to the inside the artery walls, resembling 'furring' on the inside of a kettle. When these fatty deposits harden, they form plaque which eventually causes the artery walls to lose their elasticity and obstruct blood flow. Arterial plaque can subsequently lead to blood clots, and if a coronary artery becomes completely blocked by a clot, the outcome is a heart attack.

WAYS OF HELPING

• Fish oil containing EPA (eicosapentaenoic acid) and DHA (cocosahexanoic acid) has been shown to reduce total cholesterol and triglyceride levels and decrease platelet accumulation (which can lead to blood clotting).
• Lecithin helps emulsify fat.
• Garlic prevents blood platelet stickiness and can lower cholesterol.

STROKE

A stroke entails the blood supply to part of the brain being cut off. This usually happens from a blockage in one of the cerebral arteries, or blood leaking through the walls of the blood vessels in the brain. A blood vessel haemorrhaging into the brain may also be the cause. When the brain is starved of oxygen, its tissue can die, causing loss of sensation and possible paralysis.

Of the two possible types of stroke ischaemic stroke is more common and occurs when brain ischaemia develops due to lack of blood supply to the brain. Ischaemic stroke, like heart disease, can be the result of fatty deposits on the artery walls, but in this case they build up in the arteries of the neck and head. Haemorrhagic stroke occurs when an artery leading to the brain bursts spilling blood into the brain. Although less common, this type of stroke is more likely to be fatal. It is usually caused by a weak spot in the arterial wall and typically occurs in people with high blood pressure or atherosclerosis.

People with heart disease are more at risk of having a stroke or developing thrombosis (a blood clot), but nevertheless can reduce the likelihood of either by living a healthier life. Factors which can increase the risk of stroke are: high blood pressure, smoking, atherosclerosis and age. The symptoms of a stroke are headache, dizziness, visual impairment, slurred speech and, in some cases, difficulty in swallowing.

WAYS OF HELPING

Although there are no easy ways to prevent a stroke research is being done into ways of reducing its likelihood. One unlikely source of protection may be walnuts, which contain the fatty acid alpha-linolenic acid, also present in vegetable oils like soya bean and canola. However the results are not yet conclusive.

Respiratory

FUNCTION

The respiratory system is responsible for taking in oxygen and giving off carbon dioxide by means of inhalation and exhalation.

As we age our lungs lose some of their elasticity gradually impairing breathing and affecting the gaseous exchange. The lungs become vulnerable to bacterial build-up, which can make older people prone to chest infections.

Within the respiratory system, air which enters the nose or mouth passes through the pharynx, the larynx (voice-box) and on to the trachea (windpipe). From here it passes into the lungs, situated in the upper chest, via two tubes called the bronchi. Each bronchus divides a number of times into bronchioles and end in little branches of hollow sacs called alveoli which fill with air as you breathe.

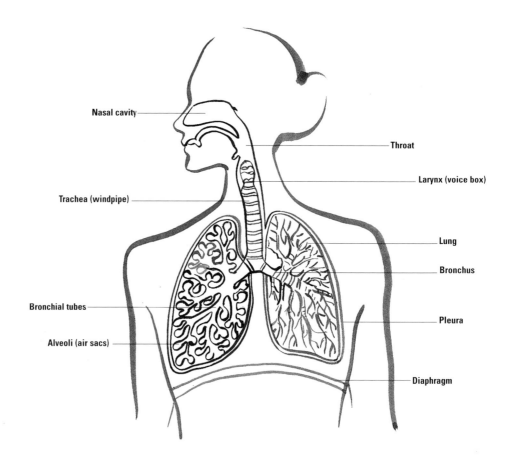

Nasal cavity

Throat

Larynx (voice box)

Trachea (windpipe)

Lung

Bronchus

Bronchial tubes

Pleura

Alveoli (air sacs)

Diaphragm

Oxygen is necessary to keep the body alive. Having been absorbed by the lungs, it is carried via the bloodstream into the cells. Here energy is released which increases the cells' ability to function. On production of energy the cells generate carbon dioxide, a waste gas which the body has no need for. The lungs remove this together with some water from the body as you breathe out. Ideally it is better to breathe in through the nose and out through the mouth. If you breathe in through the nose, the air is cleaned by the tiny hairs in the nostrils before travelling on to the throat.

Non-smokers are exposed to pollution in a smoke-filled room, and this has been linked to a variety of respiratory diseases, including lung cancer, and a greater risk of heart disease. Through inhalation of tobacco smoke, less oxygen and more carbon monoxide may be taken into the lungs.

Conditions which can affect the respiratory system include: bronchitis, pneumonia, asthma, sinusitis, emphysema and throat problems.

ASTHMA

Asthma is a condition in which the smooth muscles in the bronchioles go into spasm, causing breathing difficulties and wheezing on exhalation. There are many factors associated with asthma, both hereditary and environmental. Allergies to pollen, animal hair, feathers, dust, or fungi can bring on an attack, as can stress or anxiety. Asthma often starts in childhood or adolescence, but can equally cause problems in later life, especially after recurrent chest infections. Undeniably, cases of asthma, particularly in our cities do seem to be on the increase. Rise in pollution, particularly in the carbon monoxide fumes emitted by cars is blamed and research is currently being done on the possible long-term effects of this for asthma.

Although there is no 'cure' for the condition, there are many ways of alleviating the symptoms and reducing the number of attacks. It has been known to be brought on by acetyl salicylate, a substance found in aspirin, so if there is an allergy to acetyl salicylate, asthma sufferers should try to avoid aspirin.

WAYS OF HELPING

• Use an ionizer to clear the air of negative ions and ease breathing.
• Camomile as a tea or in a massage oil blend is anti-inflammatory and calming.
• Inhale eucalyptus oil.
• Increase vitamin C intake. Research has shown it can lower the histamine level in the blood, which is one of the causes of allergic reactions.
• Gingko biloba may help with the inflammatory side of asthma.
• Practise breathing and relaxation techniques (see chapter two) daily.
• Reflexology and acupuncture (see pages 138 and 140) may also help.

WAYS OF HELPING

• Avoid exposure to cold and damp.

• Use garlic which is anti-bacterial.

• Try essential oils of eucalyptus and camphor which contain decongestant, expectorant and anti-microbial properties. Use a couple of drops of each in the bath, as a massage oil, in a vaporizer or for a steam inhalation.

• Exercise regularly.

• Take vitamin C and echinacea which can help boost the immune system.

• Try reflexology or acupuncture s(see pages 138 and 140).

WAYS OF HELPING

• Inhale the steam from eucalyptus or peppermint oil in hot water or drops on a tissue.

• Sleep with bedhead slightly raised.

• Shiatsu on certain pressure points on the feet and hands may be beneficial (see pages 134 and 135).

BRONCHITIS

Bronchitis is caused by inflammation of the bronchi, the two airways which carry air from the windpipe to the lungs. Two forms of the disease are recognized – 'acute' where the attack is quite sudden and is only temporary, and 'chronic' where the condition is more prolonged and recurs over several years.

Acute bronchitis is usually associated with a viral infection such as influenza. Smoke inhalation and chemical pollutants can precipitate the condition, so avoid smoky atmospheres as well as dry or overheated rooms

Chronic bronchitis is due to the overproduction of mucus which begins to line the bronchi and can only be moved by coughing. Dairy products will exacerbate this. The symptoms are usually wheezing, a persistent cough with mucus, shortness of breath and sometimes chest pain and headache. Smokers, babies and the elderly are most at risk of bronchitis because of the fragility of their immune systems and lungs.

SINUSITIS

Sinuses are the air-filled spaces in the bones around the nose, eyes and cheeks. They are lined with mucous membranes, which can become inflamed, resulting in sinusitis. It is usually brought on by a cold, bacterial infection, hayfever or allergy to dust or irritants such as tobacco smoke. Symptoms are usually pain around the forehead and cheek areas, nasal congestion, loss of the sense of smell and headaches.

EMPHYSEMA

Emphysema is a condition in which the alveoli become distended and eventually destroyed as their walls collapse. Most cases of emphysema are linked to chronic bronchitis, asthma or smoking. Due to a reduction in blood flow to and from the lungs, the heart has to work harder for the circulation to function properly, which can consequently lead to heart failure because of the added strain.

The main symptoms are breathlessness, possible coughing and wheezing and blueness of the lips.

PNEUMONIA

Pneumonia is inflammation of the lungs due to infection mainly brought on by viruses or bacteria. One or both lungs can become inflamed and early symptoms are usually a cough and shortness of breath. Pneumonia is not a single disease, but a generic name for various types of lung inflammation. It can affect children and adults, but tends to be more common in males especially when elderly.

Broncopneumonia often affects both lungs and produces large amounts of green or yellow phlegm during coughing. It can be related to smoking or influenza and mainly affects the elderly. As in the case of bronchitis, it is best to avoid or reduce your consumption of dairy products as they may contribute towards a mucus build-up and congestion in the chest. To stimulate the immune system, increase your intake of garlic, vitamin C and echinacea,

Mild pneumonia can usually be treated at home, but hospitalization is necessary in more severe cases.

WAYS OF HELPING

• Give up smoking and avoid smoky or polluted atmospheres.
• Some naturopathic practitioners believe that vitamin A can strengthen the lung tissue.

SORE THROAT

Sore throat is a very common problem and usually happens for a number of reasons, though the main cause is a low resistance to infection and an impaired immune system which worsens with age. The throat is often the first area of the body to respond to viral or bacterial infection and is therefore useful in giving early warning of the impending development of a cold, laryngitis, pharyngitis or tonsillitis, or chicken pox, measles and mumps in children. In the case of tonsillitis it is often accompanied by fever and a difficulty in swallowing. With pharyngitis and laryngitis there is often either loss of voice or husky voice.

Resistance to infection can be reduced by tiredness, smoking and an unhealthy diet. Stress often manifests itself in the throat area and it is interesting that in her book *You Can Heal Your Life* Louise Hay wrote that throat problems are often found in people who find it difficult to express themselves verbally, have a build-up of anger and find it hard to say 'no'.

WAYS OF HELPING

• Avoid sugar as it only irritates the throat.
• Gargle with salt water or two or three drops of tea tree oil in water. Tea tree has remarkable anti-fungal and anti-bacterial properties.
• Suck zinc lozenges, available from most health-food shops.
• Increase your vitamin C intake together with echinacea.
• Steam inhalations with eucalyptus, benzoin and sandalwood can be beneficial.

Reproductive

FUNCTION

The main function of the female reproductive system is ovulation (the production of eggs) and the possibility of childbirth. The organs, which lie within the pelvic cavity, consist of:

- **The uterus (womb).**
- **The cervix (neck of the womb).**
- **The vagina.**
- **Two ovaries.**
- **Two Fallopian tubes.**
- **The vulva (external genitalia).**

Each month an ovum (egg) from one of the ovaries travels along the Fallopian tube leading from that ovary. If, during its journey, it is fertilized by a sperm, it will begin to divide and then embed into the lining of the uterus for development into an embryo. If fertilization does not occur, the endometrium (lining of the uterus) is shed with the help of uterine contractions. The menstrual period then begins. Women are born with around 40,000 egg cells in the ovaries, which is their lifetime supply.

Common disorders of the female reproductive system include: menorrhagia, dysmenhorrea, pre-menstrual tension, fibroids, endometriosis and thrush.

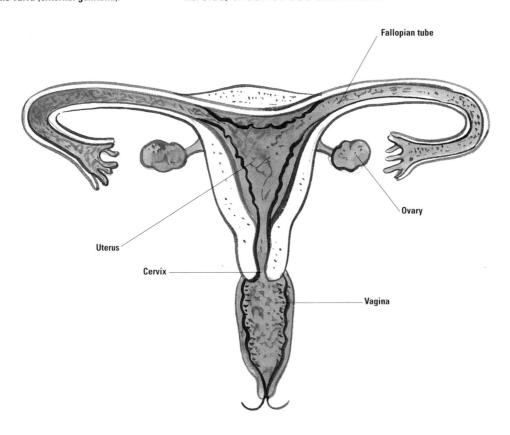

Fallopian tube

Ovary

Uterus

Cervix

Vagina

MENORRHAGIA

Menorrhagia is the term for heavy menstrual flow. Some women have naturally heavier periods than others and there are a number of possible causes. These include the presence of an IUD, small non-cancerous growths in the womb known as fibroids, cervical or endometrical polyps, ovarian cysts, uterine infection, pelvic inflammatory disease and thyroid imbalances.

Because it involves prolonged loss of blood menorrhagia often precipitates anaemia, which can be confirmed with a blood test. Hypothyroidism (underactive thyroid gland) can also cause menstrual problems as the thyroid has a hormonal influence on the ovaries, for which reason it is often called the third ovary.

WAYS OF HELPING

• Eat iron-rich foods such as liver, fish, brewer's yeast (except where yeast intolerance), prunes, egg yolks, spinach and leafy green vegetables.
• Choose amino chelated iron supplements which avoid constipation.
• Vitex agnus castus herb works on the female hormonal system (see chapter five).
• Add rose and geranium oil to a base oil, to massage stomach and back.

DYSMENORRHOEA

It really isn't necessary to suffer dysmenorrhoea (painful periods) month after month. The important factor is to determine the underlying cause, which might be fibroids, pelvic inflammatory disease, endometriosis or an IUD. Symptoms are usually cramping pains in the lower abdominal or lower back areas, nausea and sometimes a feeling of faintness.

WAYS OF HELPING

• Ease pain by lying on your back with your knees pulled up to your chest.
• Avoid caffeine to lessen tension.
• Take gentle exercise such as swimming or stretching. This increases endorphins, natural painkillers.

ENDOMETRIOSIS

Endometriosis is a condition in which particles of the endometrium (lining of the uterus) are found in other parts of the body, mainly in the pelvic area. It generally occurs in women between the ages of 20 and 40 and can sometimes cause infertility. Unfortunately the endometrial particles are not shed with the normal menstrual flow, but instead travel upwards and into the Fallopian tubes. However, they still continue to bleed monthly and can eventually cause the growth of cysts. The continual swelling of these cysts accounts for the pain associated with endometriosis.

Symptoms are usually heavy or abnormal periods, and abdominal or lower back pain during menstruation. Digestive problems can arise, such as diarrhoea, constipation and painful defaecation. Severe cases may require removal of the ovaries.

WAYS OF HELPING

• Both reflexology and acupuncture (see pages 138 and 140) work well on female reproductive problems.
• Herbs which can be beneficial include: blue cohash, a mildly stimulating uterine tonic; black cohash, which warms and stimulates the uterus and can relieve pain; and false unicorn root, which can have an oestrogenic effect.

WAYS OF HELPING

• Reflexology and acupuncture (see pages 138 and 140) can be beneficial.

• If anaemia results from heavy periods, increase your intake of iron in food or with supplements (the amino chelated variety is more readily absorbed and therefore less likely to cause constipation).

• Make sure that you have enough vitamin C in your diet to assist the absorption of iron.

FIBROIDS

A fibroid is a growth which can develop within or from the wall of the uterus and is nearly always benign. It may be as small as a pea or as large as a grapefruit. Fibroids appear most commonly in women between the ages of 35 and 45. Although the exact cause is unknown, it is thought that oestrogen can play a part as women taking oestrogen contraceptive pills sometimes have a tendency to enlarged fibroids, as do pregnant women. Post-menopausal women, whose levels of oestrogen have diminished, often experience a shrinkage in fibroids, a fact which supports the theory of oestrogen as the cause. Since body fat also produces oestrogen independent of the ovaries it is wise to reduce the risk of any excess by maintaining a reasonable weight.

Small fibroids can sometimes go unnoticed as often there are no symptoms, but in cases of larger fibroids there can be heavy or prolonged periods, blood clots, cramping pains and abdominal distension. Fibroids can also press on the bladder, resulting in the need to urinate frequently, or on the bowel, causing constipation and backache.

An ultra-sound scan of the womb enables fibroids to be viewed to confirm their size and condition. This can be carried out abdominally or vaginally, is completely painless and takes about fifteen minutes. A more recent procedure, which allows the gynaecologist to look directly into the womb is a hysteroscopy. Under anaesthetic a small instrument (about 1cm/½in diameter) called a hysteroscope, is inserted into the womb via the cervix. The gynaecologist can see whether heavy periods are caused by small fibroids growing into the uterine cavity or by very small polyps which can result in similar menstrual problems. Hysteroscopy can be carried out on an out-patient basis.

If symptoms persist, a myomectomy (an operation to remove the fibroids only) will be performed. If there are large numbers of fibroids present, a hysterectomy (removal of the womb) may be suggested. These are currently two options for problem fibroids but less invasive procedures are becoming available.

Ovarian cysts

Ovarian cysts are abnormal fluid filled swellings in an ovary. They can develop on one or both ovaries in women of any age. They are extremely common and in the majority of cases, benign or non-cancerous.

There are various different types of ovarian cysts. The most common is a follicular cyst in which the graafian follicle enlarges and fills with fluid. Another type is a corpus luteum cyst which develops if the corpus luteum (a small yellowish structure formed from the follicle after ovulation) continues to grow after the egg is released. Both follicular and corpus luteum cysts are known as functional cysts and they usually disappear on their own during the course of one or two menstrual cycles.

Cystadenomas, which are benign tumours containing fluid filled cysts together with some tissue, are also fairly common. In a few rare cases ovarian cystadenomas have become cancerous.

Dermoid cysts are also benign tumours with a cell structure similar to that of the skin, and they sometimes contain small fragments of bone and cartilage. Although they are considered harmless, your doctor will probably advise that they be removed surgically.

There are often no symptoms from ovarian cysts, but occasionally they can cause abdominal pain and menstrual problems such as delayed, heavy or painful periods. If a cyst becomes twisted or ruptured, severe abdominal pain, nausea and fever may develop.

It is important particularly in older women that an ovarian cyst is distinguished from ovarian cancer. A cyst will usually be revealed by a pelvic examination and then ultrasound scanning either abdominally or vaginally, or a laparoscopy can be carried out to confirm its size and position of the cyst. Depending on the size and nature of ovarian cysts, a cystectomy (surgical removal of a cyst) may be required. In rare cases very large ovarian cysts require an oophorectomy which is the surgical removal of the affected ovary.

WAYS OF HELPING

• Avoid wearing nylon underwear and tights, wear cotton instead.

• Avoid wearing tight clothing.

• Avoid perfumed soaps, talc or bath preparations and vaginal deodorants.

• Add tea tree oil to the bath.

• Avoid antibiotics but if taking a course, eat natural yoghurt and supplement with acidophilus bifidus.

• Always wipe from front to back after using the toilet.

• Reduce sugar and alcohol intake.

THRUSH

Thrush is the common name for candidiasis, an infection by the fungus *candida albicans*, a yeast-like organism which thrives in warm moist areas such as the throat, vagina and vulva. A certain amount of candida is normal within the body, but sometimes its growth can get out of control, usually due to overuse of antibiotics or a low-functioning immune system which has impaired resistance to infection. The growth of candida can increase with diabetes mellitus during pregnancy and with hormonal changes due to long-term use of the contraceptive pill. The symptoms of vaginal thrush are usually itching and soreness around the vaginal area, a thick white discharge and occasional discomfort during urination.

TOXIC SHOCK SYNDROME

Toxic shock syndrome (TSS) is a rare though acute illness caused by an overgrowth of the bacteria staphyloccus aureus in the vagina. First recognized in the late 1970s, it was linked to the use of tampons, particularly the highly absorbent brands which contained certain materials such as polyester foam and polyacrylate rayon. These particular brands of tampon have now been removed from the market. However, TSS still occurs in a small percentage of women, and although others of these cases are attributed to the use of tampons there are some which have been linked to the use of contraceptives such as the cap, diaphragm and sponge.

The onset of TSS is often rather quick, with symptoms such as high fever, headache, diarrhoea and vomiting, muscular aches and pains, bloodshot eyes and dizziness. These are often mistaken for flu, but sometimes a rash similar to sunburn develops on the palms of the hands and soles of the feet. These early symptoms can occasionally lead to other more serious complaints, such as a severe drop in blood pressure, and kidney, liver and perhaps lung problems.

TSS is usually treated with antibiotics and women who have had the condition are usually advised not to use tampons or contraceptive caps, diaphragms or sponges.

SELF-EXAMINATION OF THE BREASTS

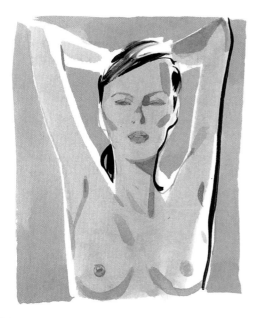

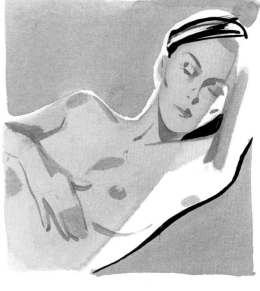

❶ Raising both arms above your head, face the mirror in a good light. Look for any changes in the shape of and size of each breast and nipple.

❷ Lie on your back with a pillow under your left shoulder blade and your head on your left arm. Squeeze the left nipple to check for discharge.

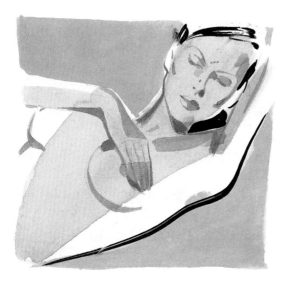

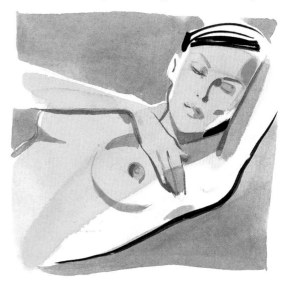

❸ With the flat of your hand, work around your left breast in small circles moving in towards the nipple. Feel for any unusual density and lumps.

❹ Be sure to check the whole armpit area, where the lymph glands are found. Press gently, moving your fingers down towards the breast.

SELF-EXAMINATION
OF THE BREASTS

On self-examination cancerous lumps will usually feel hard but painless and more often appear near the armpit at the top of the breast. Raising the arms can be a good way of detecting any change. It is best to examine yourself monthly and after a period, without clothes on, using the procedure described on page 57 for both breasts.

BREAST CANCER

Breast cancer is the most common of all the female cancers and each year thousands of new cases are diagnosed. Regular self-examination is essential in the battle against this disease. Breast lumps vary in size and shape and may be cancerous, but could be a cyst, fybroadenoma (a thickening of tissue) or a benign tumour. Breasts respond to the hormonal changes during the menstrual cycle so can feel lumpier at certain times of the month. Breast texture becomes softer as you grow older. Breast cancer is rare in young women unless there is a family history and research continues into genetic links. Long-term use of oral contraceptives and HRT have also been implicated.

After the age of 50 women are offered a mammogram (breast X-ray) up into their 70s as they are most vulnerable to the disease during this time. Most cases are treated by a lumpectomy (an operation to remove the cancerous lump only) or a mastectomy (removal of the breast).

The Imperial Cancer Research Fund is developing laser treatment to kill the tumour while causing far less damage to surrounding healthy tissue than conventional surgery.

CERVICAL CANCER

Pre-cancerous changes in the cervix are easily detected with a cervical smear test and as there are few symptoms in the early stages regular tests are vital. A colposcopy (internal inspection using a viewing instrument) can also be used for diagnosis. Sometimes cervical cancer can occur through infection from a certain organism in a male sexual partner. Genital warts in a male is another contributory factor. In these cases barrier contraceptive methods are advisable.

In recent years there have been media reports of incorrect smear test results, which have obviously caused much concern and many problems. However, a team of doctors in Australia has developed a computer-aided device which produces results within minutes, so far proving over 90 per cent correct in its diagnosis of 2,000 women. Until this test becomes available in the UK it is essential that regular smear tests are carried out.

PRE-MENSTRUAL TENSION

Unfortunately there is no way of measuring pre-menstrual tension (PMT) as no physical characteristics are apparent. This condition can be torture for some women and should be treated sympathetically. It has always existed, but until recently was never discussed. Like all women's problems it has been viewed as something which should be neither seen nor heard about. Our twentieth-century diet and environment have possibly worsened the symptoms, as they tend to be exacerbated by the usual culprits of caffeine, sugar, salt, and saturated fats, all of which often make up too high a proportion of our diet.

It is the many hormonal changes which occur between ovulation and the following menstrual period which are the cause of symptoms associated with PMT, such as swollen breasts, bloated abdomen, irritability, depression, mood swings, food cravings, headaches, skin problems, water retention and insomnia. Some women may experience none of these symptoms while others may suffer with all of them, and PMT can vary in each individual from month to month.

WAYS OF HELPING
- Take regular exercise.
- Increase your intake of calcium.
- If sugar cravings are bad, chromium-rich foods such as shellfish, nuts, grape juice, chicken, fruit and mushrooms can be beneficial. Or take chromium picolinate supplement.
- Vitex agnus castus herb can have an effect on the pituitary gland and stimulate progesterone action.
- Bach's Rescue Remedy may also be helpful (see page 109).

HERPES

Genital herpes, usually caused by the herpes simplex type II virus, is a common infection symptomized by small fluid-filled blisters. The majority of herpes simplex infections are only mildly irritating – it is the herpes simplex type I that normally causes cold sores to appear round the mouth and can also cause genital herpes. The blisters are usually small and occur in groups in the vaginal or anal area, and can be painful and itchy. Eventually the blisters burst, leaving an open sore. Attacks are more likely during pregnancy or menstruation, after sunbathing, or during times of stress and when one is generally run down.

Herpes will usually clear up in a couple of weeks even if it is untreated, but care should be taken as it is extremely contagious and genital herpes in a pregnant mother can infect her baby during its passage through the birth canal.

WAYS OF HELPING
- Avoid direct contact with the sores.
- Avoid sexual contact with an infected person.
- Wear cotton underwear.
- Dab a little lavender or tea tree oil directly on to the sores to soothe them.
- Take the amino acid lysine, as a supplement, to help control outbreaks.
- Avoid the amino acid arginine found in foods such as chocolate, carob, oats, peanuts, wheatgerm, soya beans and gelatine.

RISK FACTORS

There is no reason why a later pregnancy should not be successful, but older mothers should be aware of the risks involved:

• High blood pressure, diabetes or heart disease which are more prevalent with age can increase complications during pregnancy.

• Chromosomal abnormalities such as Down's syndrome, and conditions like spina bifida are more prevalent. At age 38 one out of 170 women gives birth to a Down's syndrome baby, increasing to one in 30 women by the age of 45.

• There is a slightly greater risk in older women of miscarriage or premature birth.

• Some studies have found a higher incidence of complications during labour and consequently greater likelihood of a caesarean delivery.

• Older mothers have a higher risk of delivering low birth-weight babies, usually as a result of decreased uterine growth.

PREGNANCY IN LATER LIFE

Many women are opting for late motherhood nowadays and there are numerous reasons for this. They may not have been in a stable relationship earlier, they may have married later, they may have needed to establish a certain career before having children, there may have been fertility problems, or, of course their pregnancy may have come as a complete surprise. Some women who may even be grandmothers seem to experience an increase in fertility around the age of 40. There are other women who decide to have a child even as a single parent.

Although there are risks, an older mother, who is fit and in good health will have gained self-awareness and experience invaluable for birth and motherhood and may even be better suited for pregnancy than someone younger in worse health.

Tests in later pregnancy

Most women over the age of 35 will automatically be offered ante-natal screening for Down's syndrome and other defects. Amniocentis and chorionic villus sampling are the two main ones available, but you can also opt for the non invasive methods of blood testing and ultra-sound. If a test reveals foetal abnormality, the option of terminating the pregnancy is offered, together with genetic counselling.

Amniocentesis entails removing a small quantity of the amniotic fluid, which surrounds the foetus, for chromosomal examination. It is normally performed between the sixteenth and twentieth week of pregnancy. The procedure usually takes about five minutes and involves the insertion of a thin needle, about 9cm/3½in long, through the abdomen and wall of the uterus, into the amniotic sac. Fluid is drawn off using a syringe which is attached to the needle. The fluid sample is then sent to a laboratory for analysis, where the results can take anything from two to six weeks. The test has been associated with miscarriage, but the risk is small. It a reliable test for Down's syndrome, but it will not determine the severity of abnormality. Nor at this stage will other problems which can arise as a result of non-genetic causes be detected.

Chorionic villus sampling enables an earlier diagnosis to be made of an abnormal foetus between nine and 12 weeks. However, unlike amniocentesis, it is unable to detect neural tube defects. Chorionic villi are the microscopic finger-like projections surrounding the chorion, the outermost membrane of the fertilized egg, which will develop into the placenta.

During the test a small catheter is inserted into the chorionic tissue, through either the abdomen or vagina, and some of the chorionic villi are drawn out. The chorionic villi cells are then grown in a special culture in preparation for analysis. The procedure takes about half an hour and the results are available in two to four weeks, sometimes less. The advantage with CVS is that if there is an abnormality in the foetus and the parents decide to terminate the pregnancy, this can be carried out earlier than with amniocentesis.

Material blood bio-chemistry testing is also known as the triple test, Leeds or Bart's test. Introduced by St Bartholomew's Hospital Medical College in London, it enables a more precise estimate to be given of the risk of Down's Syndrome. The test involves taking 10ml of blood from the mother at 15 weeks of the pregnancy onwards and measuring two hormones (oestriol, a form of oestrogen, and HCG, a human chorionic gonadotrophin) and one protein (alpha-fetoprotein). If the risk is at the unacceptably high level for the couple, an amniocentesis or CVS would be recommended to exclude a chance of chromosomal abnormality.

Detailed ultra-sound examination is performed by an expert at 20 weeks to diagnose physical defects which may or may not be due to chromosomal abnormalities.Ultrasound is safe, but not infallible.

It is important to realize that all non-invasive tests still involve risk factors to the child whether there are chromosomal abnormalities or not. The woman's age is taken into consideration and then afterwards she can decide whether to go on to have invasive testing. The advantage of an invasive test is that it gives you a definite answer. The disadvantage is, however small it may be, there is a chance of miscarriage.

WAYS OF HELPING

• **Have regular sexual intercourse.**

• **After intercourse lie with a pillow supporting the pelvic area for about 20 minutes, to help the sperm to move upwards towards the Fallopian tubes.**

• **Avoid smoking, a high alcohol intake, excessive exercise, obesity, too much caffeine, recreational drugs and stress.**

• **Include adequate protein in your diet, especially vegetable protein, as it is essential for egg production.**

• **B vitamins are important for fertility, early embryonic development and hormonal development.**

• **Polyunsaturated oils are vital for healthy sperm and the functioning of the female reproductive cycle.**

• **Vitamin E may increase fertility.**

• **Zinc and magnesium are important for healthy sperm and egg production.**

• **Supplements of the amino acid arginine together with zinc may raise sperm count in infertile men, as may the Saw Palmetto herb.**

INFERTILITY

Infertility is the inability or difficulty in conceiving a baby. Most women naturally assume from an early age that they will be able to have children of their own, but unfortunately for some couples becoming pregnant can turn into a major life crisis. Psychologically, for certain women, infertility can create a feeling of impaired femininity because they see it as an essential part of womanhood. It can be a devastating and frustrating experience for both partners creating a feeling of total failure and possible isolation.

Infertility can put a terrible strain on a relationship and it is important not to place too much emphasis on whichever partner has the physiological problem. After all, both partners share the psychological pain of so desperately wanting a child. Communication, love and support are vital for couples suffering the anguish of infertility and it is during these times that a strong bond between a couple needs to be maintained, as there is often pressure from family and friends who may be unaware of the situation.

Infertility is usually determined by a doctor after an assessment which is carried out on both partners who have been trying for a baby for twelve months or more. This is because 80-90 per cent of couples can expect to conceive within a year, although others may conceive within one to six months. Full medical and family histories are taken into consideration, and a male sperm count test is carried out at an early stage as problems in this area could delay the more complicated tests necessary for detecting problems concerning the woman.

One of the easiest initial checks that should be made is that you are ovulating. A urine testing kit measures the luteinizing hormone (LH) which rises rapidly just before ovulation or take your temperature before getting out of bed in the morning. The basal body temperature test can be done using a special thermometer available from most chemists, or a digital one. When ovulating, the temperature rises by around 0.2-0.5°C/ 0.5-1°F, generally around days 14 to 16 of the cycle.

CAUSES OF INFERTILITY

These are the possible causes of infertility in both men and women.

FAILURE TO OVULATE

Some women fail to ovulate, or ovulate very infrequently. There are various reasons for this, such as an undiagnosed hormonal imbalance, an ovarian problem such as cysts, pronounced weight loss and even stress or anxiety.

BLOCKED FALLOPIAN TUBES

Sometimes an infection can cause a blockage, thus closing the passageway for sperm, and preventing conception.

FIBROIDS

These non-malignant tumours in the womb sometimes prevent the fertilized egg from successful implantation.

ENDOMETRIOSIS

Pieces of tissue which normally line the womb begin to grow around the Fallopian tubes or ovaries and this will affect the chance of conception.

LACK OF PROGESTERONE

Progesterone normally prepares the womb for a possible egg implantation. If too little of this hormone is secreted, implantation fails to occur.

CERVICAL MUCUS PROBLEMS

During ovulation cervical mucus normally becomes thinner to enable the sperm to pass through more easily. Sometimes the mucus remains thick, preventing the passage of sperm through the cervix, and in rare cases it may contain certain antibodies which can destroy the sperm.

PROLONGED USE OF AN INTRAUTERINE DEVICE (IUD)

Complications sometimes associated with an IUD, such as pelvic inflammatory disease and uterine perforation, can reduce a woman's chances of becoming pregnant.

OVERSTRENUOUS EXERCISE AND EXCESSIVE DIETING

These can affect ovulation as secretion of the reproductive hormones such as oestrogen are affected when excess weight is lost.

DRUG ABUSE

Controlled drugs and narcotics can alter the secretion of certain hormones as well as affecting the movement of sperm and the health of women's eggs.

LOW SPERM COUNT

Male sperm count has dropped by 50 per cent in the last 50 years. This dramatic decline has been linked to toxic chemicals found in our water. These chemicals mimic oestrogen, a female hormone of which men naturally have a little and excess exposure to oestrogen has been shown to bring about reproductive changes in fish.

MEDICATION

Some medications can interfere with fertility.

SMOKING

Smokers usually produce fewer eggs.

EXPOSURE TO CERTAIN ENVIRONMENTAL TOXINS

Dioxins and dioxin-like PCBs are known to adversely effect the body. A recent study in the USA showed that exposure to dioxins caused female rhesus monkeys to develop endometriosis, and the greater their exposure, the greater the severity of the disease.

ADVANCING YEARS

Both men and women become less fertile with age and a woman's supply of eggs becomes very diminished once she is into her 40s.

WAYS OF TESTING INFERTILITY

To test for infertility in women one of these methods will be used.

LAPAROSCOPY AND HYSTEROSCOPY

In laparoscopy a small telescope is inserted through the naval into the abdomen to check for abnormalities like endometriosis, adhesions and blockages in the Fallopian tubes, uterus and ovaries. For a hysteroscopy, the telescope is inserted through the vagina and cervix, is sometimes carried out to view the inside of the uterus. Both are performed under general anaesthetic and usually take one or two hours.

PROGESTERONE LEVEL BLOOD TEST

A progesterone level blood test is usually carried out on the twentieth or twenty-first day of the monthly cycle. Progesterone levels should rise after ovulation in preparation for a fertilized egg. Low levels can signify an underdeveloped endometrial lining, making implantation of an egg impossible.

ENDOMETRIAL BIOPSY

Endometrial biopsy can be carried out without anaesthesia. A sample of uterine tissue is removed surgically after the twenty-first day of the monthly cycle. It is tested for any abnormalities and to ascertain whether ovulation has taken place. Although advanced technology should make this test painless, some women find it uncomfortable, in which case a local anaesthetic may be given.

HYSTEROSALPINGOGRAM By means of a catheter a special dye is inserted into the cervix which flows into the uterus and fallopian tubes. The test is carried out about a week after menstruation and enables the specialist to see if the fallopian tubes are open and to check the interior of the uterus. There is usually some abdominal cramping during this procedure, so anti-inflammatory medication is normally suggested.

HYSTEROSALPINGO CONTRAST SONOGRAPHY

Hysterosalpingo contrast sonography (HyCoSy) allows doctors to obtain a clear image of the Fallopian tubes within 15 minutes. It uses Echovist, a solution containing tiny bubbles which glow around the outside of the fallopian tubes. Using transvaginal ultra-sound the images show any blockages or abnormal functioning within the Fallopian tubes. HyCoSy requires no hospital stay or anaesthetic, it is carried out in the outpatients department and takes about 30 minutes.

POST-COITAL TEST

A post-coital test looks at the woman's cervical mucus and also the sperm's interaction with it. It has to be carried out within a few hours of sexual intercourse, prior to or during ovulation. The cervical mucus is removed with a syringe, and if it is normal, actively moving sperm should be visible.

INFERTILITY TREATMENT

All these treatments cost a lot financially and emotionally, but with increasing technology the possibility of achieving pregnancy is improving. If a man and a woman both eat a healthy diet, exercise moderately, get enough sleep and enjoy a healthy sex life, they will be doing the best they can to help natural conception and, where necessary, to assist their fertility programme.

ARTIFICIAL INSEMINATION

Artifical insemination is a way of introducing semen into the woman's cervix using a small syringe and is generally used in cases where a woman's partner is infertile or subfertile, or where there are sexual, psychological or physical difficulties. The process can use either the husband's semen or that of a donor. Insemination using the husband's semen is usually carried out in cases of low sperm count or physical or sexual difficulties. Donor insemination is normally carried out if the husband is infertile or there are genetic problems, and the donor usually remains anonymous. Semen from a donor is frozen and stored after tests to ensure that it contains no dangerous micro-organisms. The semen is depositied directly into the woman's cervix during her ovulating days and is usually repeated on a monthly basis for about six months unless a pregnancy occurs.

IN VITRO FERTILIZATION

In vitro literally means 'in glass' and describes the petri dish in which a woman's eggs are placed after removal from her ovaries. Prior to treatment a woman is given fertility drugs to assist the ripening of her eggs. This is monitored during the next four or five days using an ultra-sound scan. Ripe eggs are removed either by laparoscopy or an ultra-sound guided needle through the abdomen or vagina. They are then mixed with the husband's sperm in the petri dish, and incubated for about two days. The eggs are examined to see if fertilization has occurred and embryo development has begun and if so, a few fertilized eggs are removed to be placed back into the uterus via the vagina. In vitro fertilization (IVF) is often used in cases of blocked or missing Fallopian tubes, or if the woman's cervical mucus is incompatible with her partner's sperm.

GAMETE INTRAFALLOPIAN TRANSFER

Gamete intrafallopian transfer (Gift) is used when the woman's fallopian tubes are not obstructed. The ovaries are first activated by certain drugs, then fluid is sucked out from the ovarian follicles through a needle by means of a laparoscopy under general anaesthesia. After the fluid has been examined under a microscope for eggs, these and the partner's sperm (gametes) are inserted together into the Fallopian tubes where, it is hoped, fertilization will happen.

ZYGOTE INTRAFALLOPIAN TRANSFER (ZIFT)

Zygote intrafallopian transfer (Zift) is a similar procedure to IVF treatment in that the eggs and sperm are combined in a petri dish and incubated for two days. The difference is that fertilization of the eggs is confirmed prior to being placed into the Fallopian tubes, from where they then travel the normal route into the uterus for implantation.

WAYS OF HELPING

• For a prolapsed uterus, practise the pelvic floor muscles on page 43.

• Reflexology and acupuncture can be helpful (see pages 138 and 140).

• Vitamin C and E will aid internal healing post-operatively.

• Take arnica which reduces bruising and swelling before and after the operation to assist post-operative recovery.

For details of individual support groups in your area contact Women's Health (see page 218).

HYSTERECTOMY

Hysterectomy (removal of the uterus) is a common operation in the UK. A total hysterectomy removes both the uterus and the cervix. In some cases the ovaries and Fallopian tubes are also removed, especially where there is a chance of ovarian cancer. Generally, however, removal of the ovaries is unnecessary, especially in pre-menopausal women. If the ovaries are removed, the likelihood of bone fractures in later life may be increased through lack of oestrogen leading to osteoporosis. Nowadays a transcervical resection of the endometrium (TCRE) may be performed as an alternative to hysterectomy for women with heavy bleeding.

The purpose of hysterectomy is usually the treatment of problematic fibroids, and uterine or cervical cancer. It can also be performed in cases of severe menorrhagia, endometriosis and acute prolapsed uterus. The operation is carried out abdominally or vaginally.

Whichever form of hysterectomy is carried out, total or partial, it is still major surgery which should be avoided if at all possible. Cancer is the exception. Contrary to many orthodox ways of thinking the uterus is more than just a vessel for a growing foetus, and its removal is not a cure-all for gynaecological problems. In fact the sudden loss of oestrogen can precipitate various problems, apart from osteoporosis, that a woman would not usually expect for perhaps at least another ten years, such as heart disease, incontinence and other symptoms associated with ageing and the menopause.

For some women hysterectomy can also seem like the loss of femininity as the womb is not just a reproductive organ but also a very important part of the body. Removing it can cause a deep sense of loss and anxiety. It is therefore very important to discuss the issue with both your partner and gynaecologist before making any final decision, and get a second or third opinion if in any doubt.

Recovery from a hysterectomy can take anything from two weeks to six months depending on the gravity of complications involved, and the individual's own ability to recover.

THE MENOPAUSE

The term menopause, coined in 1821 by a French physician called Gardanne, comes from the Greek *meno* meaning month and *pausis* meaning end or, more literally, a pause in a life cycle. The menopause is nature's way of ending fertility with the cessation of menstruation. Until recently the menopause was a subject that was avoided and certainly never discussed in public. After all, no one wanted to admit that they were approaching the 'beginning of the end', which is how the menopause was viewed years ago. Society saw menopausal women as old. Today there are opportunities to learn more about both the physical and mental aspects of this transition in life. For many women menopause is seen as a milestone in the ageing process and it is natural to feel a little anxious about the changes that lie ahead and their affect on physical appearance.

Menopause may mean the loss of the ability to choose to have children, but it should never mean a lost ability to choose a healthier life. How you prepare for menopause and respond to it is extremely important. Positive thinking will eradicate the negative emotions which so often accompany the menopause.

The Physiological facts

The menopause usually occurs between the ages of 45 and 55, although there are some cases of premature menopause in the 30s, sometimes as a result of the removal of the ovaries, hereditary factors or possibly heavy smoking.

Prior to the menopause the ovaries, under the influence of the pituitary gland, produce an egg approximately each month ready for fertilization. This very important gland actually governs the whole of the endocrine system by controlling the output of various hormones on a day-to-day basis. As well as the eggs, which come pre-formed as Graafian follicles, the ovaries also produce ovarian stoma or supporting tissue. It is within these two substances that the hormones oestrogen and progesterone are secreted.

During our menstruating years each month several of these follicles are stimulated monthly by a hormone from the pituitary

SYMPTOMS

Although a symptom-free menopause is not uncommon, symptoms you may experience from the withdrawal of oestrogen include:

• Hot flushes.

• Vaginal dryness.

• Night sweats.

• Changes in skin and hair condition.

• Urinary problems.

• Loss of libido.

• Depression.

gland called follicle stimulating hormone (FSH). This enables one or more follicles to grow and release an egg, usually at the mid-point of the cycle. This process is known as ovulation. A second hormone, also secreted by the pituitary gland is called the luteinizing hormone (LH), and this also plays an important part in assisting this process. As well as controlling the process of ovulation, FSH and LH control the circulation of oestrogen and progesterone.

After ovulation, oestrogen levels drop slightly and are joined by the second female hormone progesterone which prepares the lining of the womb for a possible implantation of the egg. If fertilization does not occur, the level of progesterone drops, causing the lining of the womb to shed. It is this process which brings about the monthly period.

In the lead-up to the menopause things change as basically the ovaries become tired. The Graafian follicles slowly diminish in number and oestrogen levels decrease. Consequently, to alleviate the workload of the ovaries, the pituitary gland releases more FSH. At the same time the follicles start to grow at a slower, more irregular rate increasing or decreasing the time between the cycles and causing irregular periods. As ovulation becomes erratic, progesterone levels also decrease. The pituitary gland still tries to help by secreting more LH, but in the end the lining of the womb loses its stimulus and menstrual periods eventually cease as a result of the severe drop in oestrogen levels. This marks the natural end of a woman's fertility.

For a few years afterwards levels of FSH and LH will continue to be fairly high, but eventually they will fall away. The lead-up to the menopause can take as long as five years and is divided into the pre-menopause, when periods become irregular and vary in flow, and the peri-menopause, when physical and psychological symptoms are sometimes first noticed. The years following the menopause are known as the post-menopause. As a woman's periods become very infrequent during the years leading up to menopause, it is often difficult to pinpoint until some time after the event exactly when the final one occured.

Hot flushes and night sweats Hot flushes and night sweats are the most common of all menopausal symptoms and the most visibly noticeable. They are caused partly by a withdrawal of oestrogen and are preceded by a surge in hormone activity by the hypothalmus (an area of the brain adjacent to the pituitary gland). Among the hormones released is one which elevates the level of LH from the pituitary gland. There is also increased activity in the area of the nervous system which controls blood pressure, blood flow and the adrenal glands. As the hypothalamus governs the pituitary, it is evident that these flushes are not due to a change in the sex hormones, but to effects which the pituitary incurs in the change of activity in the hypothalamus which also controls and regulates body temperature. It is apparent that the hot flush is more a 'brain' issue than a hormonal occurrence.

Hot flushes are usually felt in the face, neck and chest and sometimes the arms. The blood flow increases in the affected area, causing a redness and a rise in temperature due to expansion of the blood vessels. Sometimes this will be accompanied by sweating which acts to cool the skin. For some people hot flushes bring about an increase in blood pressure and heart rate, often causing a feeling of exhaustion and anxiety. If the flushes occur at night, the normal sleep pattern is disturbed, which can account for depression, irritability and fatigue.

WAYS OF HELPING
- Minimize hot drinks like tea and coffee which increase insomnia and anxiety.
- Avoid spicy foods.
- Avoid overheated environments.
- Give up smoking which affects the circulatory system and bone density and can bring on an early menopause.
- Wear clothes made of fabrics such as cotton that allow the skin to 'breathe'.
- Use pure cotton bed linen and avoid heavy duvets.
- Reduce your alcohol consumption.
- Increase your calcium and vitamin D intake. Boron maintains healthy bones.
- Increase your intake of essential fatty acids.
- Practise relaxation and meditation.
- Take regular exercise.

Vaginal dryness The diminished levels of oestrogen affect the tissues of the female reproductive system. Dryness occurs as the vaginal skin becomes thinner, loses elasticity, and as its secretions lessen the mucous membranes become dry and inflamed. This can cause minor infections as well as painful sexual intercourse.

WAYS OF HELPING
- Include plant oestrogens in your diet.
- Take supplements of vitamins A, C and zinc to keep vaginal membranes healthy.
- Use vaginal lubricants but avoid petroleum jelly.

Loss of libido Loss of oestrogen also affects the nervous system, thereby influencing our response to touch. This is why sexual arousal and response decreases, resulting in loss of libido. As the adrenal glands continue to produce oestrogen

WAYS OF HELPING
- Reflexology and shiatsu can help.
- Boost adrenal glands with vitamin C and panothenic acid.

during and after the menopause, it is particularly important to avoid stress which will put a strain on the adrenals.

WAYS OF HELPING
• Reduce your tea and coffee intake.
• Include plant oestrogens in your diet.
• Practise pelvic floor exercises (see page 43).

Urinary problems As the neck of the urethra undergoes similar changes to the vagina it becomes weaker and loses muscular control. Urinary frequency, urinary incontinence when coughing or sneezing and minor infections are all common occurrences during the post-menopausal stage.

Natural oestrogens

Natural oestrogens (phyto-oestrols) are compounds whose molecular structure is similar to that of oestrogen and their effects are comparable even though they are weaker than the hormone itself. They are plant-based, the richest source being soya bean products. It is interesting that in Japan, where soya is part of their daily diet, women very rarely suffer from the side effects of the menopause or PMT. In fact a study in the Lancet magazine in 1992 concluded that these women did not seem to experience hot flushes at all. Phyto-oesterols have also been used in treating other oestrogen-deficient conditions, such as infrequent, heavy and painful periods.

Phyto-oestrols can be found in soya beans, soya flour, soy sauce, tofu (soya bean curd), myso, tamari, alfalfa, celery, fennel, green and yellow vegetables and linseeds. They are also present in the following herbs dong quai, vitex agnus castus, black cohash and sage. Recent studies have shown that vitex can increase the production of luteinizing hormone and may stimulate the production of progesterone. These herbs should be taken under the guidance of a qualified herbalist.

Natural progesterones

The richest source of natural progesterone is wild yam. It contains diosgenin, which is easily converted into progesterone in the body. Progesterone is a key hormone in the manufacture of oestrogen and can have a profound effect on preventing osteoporosis. Dong quai, black cohash and fennel also contain natural progesterones.

HORMONE REPLACEMENT THERAPY

Hormone replacement therapy (HRT) is given as a means of topping up the body's oestrogen levels which have declined either during the menopause or in the years leading up to it. It is sometimes prescribed in cases where the ovaries have been removed for medical reasons.

Whatever type of oestrogen is given, most women are additionally prescribed progesterone to protect against the possible risk of uterine cancer. Obviously this does not affect women who have undergone a hysterectomy.

Different forms of HRT

There are various ways of taking Hormone replacement therapy. Different methods work for different people and it may take a while for you to find the one that suits you. Whichever one you choose, your body will need time to adapt to it.

Tablets taken by mouth daily Commonly used but may cause nausea as the HRT passes through the liver before reaching the target areas of the body. It tends to lose some of its strength after its conversion in the liver.

Vaginal cream Provides oestrogen to the vagina and vulva directly, improving lubrication. Vaginal dryness responds well to HRT as the tissue contains oestrogen receptors. This method is not usually used long-term. It does not contain enough oestrogen to protect against heart disease and osteoporosis.

Skin patches The patch, which comes in different strengths, releases a steady supply of oestrogen bypassing the liver so avoiding the nausea caused by some preparations. It should be applied twice weekly to the hip or lower abdominal area. Progesterone will also be given as a supplement for the prevention of uterine cancer for those women who have not undergone hysterectomy.

Implants Oestrogen implant placed under skin of lower abdomen. This will be effective for up to six months and can be forgotten about once inserted. Monthly progesterone is needed by women who have not undergone hysterectomy. Some women are affected by the high oestrogen level in the implant.

BENEFITS OF HRT

• Increases bone density, reducing osteoporosis and therefore the risk of bone fractures from brittle bones in post-menopausal women.

• Alleviates symptoms of the menopause such as hot flushes, night sweats, vaginal dryness.

• Lowers risk of heart disease and stroke.

SIDE EFFECTS OF HRT

There is always a risk of side effects with any medication but the most common ones associated with HRT are:

- Weight gain.
- Nausea.
- Headaches.
- Migraines.
- Breast tenderness.
- Leg cramps.
- Breakthrough bleeding (this can be altered by changing the dosage).

Contraindications

You should not take HRT if you have a history of breast, uterine or any oestrogen-dependant cancer, in cases of thrombosis, endometriosis, liver or kidney conditions, vaginal bleeding or pancreatic disease. It is also advisable to inform your doctor if a family member has suffered from any of these.

Medication can interact with HRT's efficiency, so it is advisable to have a medical check-up before deciding on HRT.

How long should HRT be taken?

The length of time for which HRT can be taken varies according to the individual. If it is prescribed for menopausal symptoms, one to five years is the usual recommendation. For osteoporosis it is often at least ten years.

It is extremely important to have regular breast screening as the risk of developing cancer of the breast increases with the duration of treatment.

HRT withdrawal

The slower the withdrawal, the better, so that the body can adapt gradually. There may be a few oestrogen-withdrawal symptoms, such as hot flushes and headaches, though these depend on the dosage previously taken.

The menopause is a natural part of life, not a disease, so the question is whether or not our hormones need to be replaced when nature obviously intended otherwise. Every woman has the right to decide for herself, and the choice is difficult when the pros and cons are considered together. At the end of the day she should base her decision on her own health history and her personal experience of the menopause. HRT is not intended as a 'cure' but simply as a means of relieving the associated symptoms. Research and trials will continue and new products will continually become available. It is time for women to take their health into their own hands: by learning about their bodies, particularly their hormonal system, and improving their diet and lifestyle they will be elevated to better health and, it is to be hoped, a symptom-free menopause.

Hair

Hair growth generally slows down from around the age of 45, sometimes earlier or later, but from then more hairs tend to be lost than are replaced. A normal daily hair loss can be anywhere between 100 and 200 hairs.

Genetic inheritance determines the structure and colour of an individual's hair, but diet and lifestyle also play a very important part in its condition. The fact that pedigree animals are given special diets and sometimes supplements to improve the condition of their coats makes this point quite clearly.

The way our hair looks has a great effect on how we feel. Like glowing skin, shiny, lustrous hair is synonymous with good health. Our hair has no blood supply or living cells as it is technically dead. Diet, age and hormones directly determine its appearance.

The greying of hair is due to the loss of natural pigment, and although a natural procedure, some women do find it distressing. In most women greying can occur at any time during the 30s and 40s.

WHAT CAN CAUSE GREYING OR HAIR LOSS

Anaemia The most important mineral content of hair is iron, so in cases of iron deficiency and anaemia, problems such as thinning and a generally dull appearance are common.

Pregnancy Pregnancy often causes temporary hair loss.

Hypothyroidism An underactive thyroid gland can contribute.

Stress Excess stress can cause both hair loss and greying.

Certain medications If you experience unaccountable hair loss, it is worth investigating the possibility of medications being responsible.

A drop in oestrogen During the menopause a drop in oestrogen can have quite profound effects on hair.

Diets Crash diets lacking in protein, can cause hair loss.

Heriditary factors Your genes and heriditary influences can play a part.

FUNCTION

We are all born with 85,000-95,000 hair follicles, which is our lifetime's supply. Any changes to our hair during this time are due to the functioning of the follicles.

WAYS OF HELPING HAIR

• Vitamins B complex and C provide nourishment for the hair follicles. Also take pantothenic acid (vitamin B5) to relieve stress and vitamin A for a dry scaly scalp.

• Biotin is thought to prevent greying.

• Massaging the scalp during shampooing helps to remove dead skin cells and increase circulation. Beneficial oils are geranium or rosemary oil to control an oily scalp, lavender or sandal-wood for a dry scalp) and tea tree or rosemary to help to control dandruff.

• The Chinese herb fo-ti (drunk as a tea) is said to help prevent greying.

• An infusion of nettles benefits dark hair or camomile for fair hair.

• Essential fatty acids promote healthy shiny hair by feeding the hair follicles.

• Silica, a mineral in the horsetail plant, can strengthen the hair.

• Inositol in lecithin, adds lustre.

• Take iron supplements if necessary.

Skin

FUNCTION

The skin is the largest eliminative organ in the human body. Its functions include:

• Regulating body temperature.

• Providing a waterproof protective covering.

• Producing vitamin D.

• Serving as an excretory organ and a sensory covering.

Our physiological health has a major effect on the condition of the skin and the appearance of the skin has a considerable psychological effect on us. Skin blemishes can cause us to feel embarrassed, particularly if they are on the face, as it is our faces which initially portray us as people. As we grow older the condition of our skin becomes even more relevant as the skin presents the most visible evidence of ageing, such as wrinkling, unevenness in pigmentation, loss of elasticity and dryness. Unfortunately society associates wrinkles with ageing and therefore we become afraid that people will regard us as 'old' if they see wrinkles. It is often that we have our life's experiences etched on our faces in a number of expression lines. Someone with lines around the eye area may have had a lot of laughter in their life, or equally they may have had a lot of sorrow. A person who has studied for long periods or had to concentrate on, say, a word processor or intricate machinery may develop frown lines. These expression lines seem to be accepted naturally in men as 'character' lines, but in women there still seems to exist the age association.

CHANGES THAT OCCUR AS WE GROW OLDER

The degeneration of an individual's skin depends greatly on genetic inheritance, but even more so on lifestyle and diet. Our predecessors may have had wonderfully youthful skins, but if we live a lifetime of eating junk food, we are not always as lucky. During our 40s our skin starts to loose its natural oil content as the sebaceous glands begin to deteriorate, making it thinner and less elastic. Our supply of collagen, which makes up a large part of the body's connective tissue, also declines. This, together with the decline in the functioning of the nerve endings and blood vessels, affects the tone, texture and process of skin renewal. Liver spots appear because of a decrease in melanolytes, the cells which produce the tanning pigment known as melanin. The decrease in oestrogen, which usually begins to happen around the age of 40 and continues through to the menopause, is another contributory factor. Loss of support to the blood vessels causes their expansion and consequently broken veins appear.

One of the easiest ways to reduce the likelihood of wrinkling is to drink more water. The body's water component is around 60-70 per cent and this constantly needs replacing as it is used for dissolving toxins and eliminating them from the body and also for the transportation of nutrients. Water is needed to replenish our cells' moisture content and a well-hydrated body will give the skin a smooth glowing look. To keep your skin healthy aim to drink 1½ -2 litres/2½ -3½ pints of water daily, preferably filtered or bottled.

FREE RADICAL DAMAGE

Free radical damage plays a large part in the ageing process of skin (see page 15). A free radical is a molecule that has lost one of its electrons which normally function in pairs. In the need to renew the balance it tries to steal a nearby electron, eventually creating a chain reaction which causes damage to the cells' DNA, protein and fats.

It is when the free radicals react with the protein molecules in the tissues or cells that they can become tangled together. This is known as 'cross-linking'. When leather is beaten, a cross-linking effect is produced: this accounts for the comparison between ageing skin and leather.

ANTI-OXIDANTS

Anti-oxidants are very important for the skin as they protect cell life and collagen and minimize cross-linking. Anti-oxidants are not a recent discovery, but the recognition of their benefits in certain medical trials has gained attention during the past few years. They should be a part of our general diet as they are also important for the body's metabolism and chemistry. Nutrients whether from food or supplements which contain anti-oxidizing properties, neutralize free radicals and can thus combat the damaging effects that lead to skin's ageing.

WAYS OF HELPING

• Give your skin the oil it needs from essential fatty acids. These improve the skin's moisture content, preventing dehydration and improving the flexibility of the skin. Sources of EFAs include oily fish, linseeds, sunflower and sesame seeds or the cold-pressed oils made from the seeds.

• Increase blood flow to the skin through exercise and massage to improve its oxygen supply.

• Give up smoking as it narrows the blood vessels starving the skin of oxygen.

• Avoid exposure to the sun. When older we produce less melanin which protects us against its harmful ultra-violet rays.

• Take supplements of zinc and vitamin B6 to assist skin repair.

• Improve your diet: feed your skin and not your cravings.

• Keep the skin well moisturized.

Teeth

Unlike our skin, which renews itself constantly, our teeth are for life, or so we hope! It is therefore essential that we eat a healthy diet and have good dental care. Good nutrition plays an important part.

Only two or three decades ago decaying teeth which had to be filled were a constant worry. Nowadays greater knowledge and technical advancements in dentistry enable people in general to retain their teeth for longer. Twenty years ago, for example, a 60-year-old would probably have had her teeth removed whereas today inlays, crowns, veneers and specialized gum treatments are a possibility. New techniques and materials are developing constantly. From the age of 40 periodontal (gum) disease is very common, causing loosening of the teeth, bleeding gums and bad breath. This, more than dental decay, is the main reason for tooth loss in humans. Gum disease is caused by the daily bacterial plaque build-up around the neck of the tooth which gets underneath the gum line. Plaque formation rapidly increases in the presence of sugar, literally during the first 30 seconds of exposure. In the USA around 9kg/20lb of sugar is consumed per person on average every year, often through the hidden sources of prepared foods and drinks.

Elderly people often start to eat sweeter foods as their taste buds decline in number and function. Salivary flow also decreases, thereby providing less protection for gums and teeth. Many of the elderly are taking long-term medication, which can frequently cause a dry mouth. Medication in the forms of syrup, lozenges and even homeopathic pills (which sometimes contain sugar and need to be dissolved slowly under the tongue) is being recognized as a problem by dentists. In the older patient tooth decay is increasing, often attacking the exposed necks of teeth and the area between the tooth enamel and fillings.

Tooth erosion is a fairly new problem too. Soft drinks and diet drinks have a high acid content which can strip the necks and tips of teeth of their enamel, thereby exposing the dentine which is very sensitive. Citrus fruits, now more readily available all year round, are also very acidic.

Loss of teeth in one part of the mouth can give rise to excessive wear of teeth elsewhere. For example, loss of a back tooth, which is common in the older generation, can cause front teeth to wear down because of the imbalance of the top and bottom jaws. Gradually they sink closer together. Folds appear at the corners of the mouth as the jaws are no longer kept apart to the original height. This can give the face a 'sunken' look. However, modern dentistry can correct this problem with impressive results. Hormonal changes in pregnant and menopausal women can affect teeth and gums, so a healthy is diet is particularly important during these times.

FLUORIDE

There are two kinds of fluoride, calcium fluoride which is a naturally occurring mineral and sodium fluoride which is added by the water companies to some drinking water supplies as it is thought to prevent tooth decay and increase bone strength (a very important factor in the formation of teeth and bones during childhood). Fluoride is beneficial in its ability to strengthen the mineral composition of the tooth enamel, making it more resistant to acid attack in the mouth. However, it is important to realize that tooth decay is not caused solely by lack of fluoride but more often by a diet high in sugar, sweets and sugar-containing drinks being the worst offenders.

Sodium fluoride is also added to certain toothpastes and mouthwashes. If levels in the water supplies are particularly low, children are sometimes given fluoride tablets or drops. Fluoride can be applied directly to the teeth by a dentist too. There has been a lot of controversy over the years concerning the enforced supplies of sodium fluoride in water and it has even been linked to some forms of cancer in the USA. Fluoridated areas have, according to some reports, been proved to have a greater incidence of cancer. The debate for and against fluoride will continue and while excessively high levels (over eight parts per million) may lead to certain degenerative conditions in health, it is unlikely that there is any concrete link between fluoride and premature death

WAYS OF HELPING

• Elderly people should be more vigilant about the sugar content of food, drinks and oral medication.

• Have regular check-ups at the dentist: every six months, or every three to six months for the elderly as a preventative measure.

• Reduce your overall sugar intake.

• Use mouthwashes with care as some can be rather acidic.

• Increase your vitamin C intake. It assists the production of collagen (essential for healthy gums) and has healing benefits.

• Co-enzyme Q10 is thought to counteract gum disease.

• Add two or three drops of tea tree oil to a glass of water and use it as a gargle. Tea tree has anti-bacterial and anti-fungal properties. Many toothpastes on the market now contain it.

• It is important for parents to teach children dental care from an early age.

Eyes

The main problems which can affect the eyes as we grow older are:

- Cataracts.
- Glaucoma.
- Macular degeneration.

As we get older our eyesight tends to deteriorate. For most people this is inconvenient rather than painful as they have to adjust to using and wearing glasses, but more serious problems can also arise.

GLAUCOMA

Glaucoma is one of the most common eye disorders in people over the age of 60. It is caused by a build-up of fluid in the eye which causes pressure on the eye and damage to the optic nerve. A simple form of glaucoma can start in the 40s when gradual loss of peripheral vision may be experienced, but this is usually symptom-free.

The symptoms of acute glaucoma are usually a dull ache in and above the eye, cloudy vision and nausea. It is sometimes hereditary, so anyone with a family history of the condition should have regular eye checks. The symptoms can be controlled if the condition is diagnosed early enough. It is best to avoid direct sunlight, glare and bright lights indoors if you have glaucoma.

CATARACTS

Cataracts are often considered to be part of the natural ageing process. They occur as a result of protein fibres within the lens of the eye which cause opacity or lack of transparency obscuring vision. They are more common in people over 70 and can be corrected with surgery. Sometimes they can begin to form earlier on in life, especially where there has been injury to the eye or chemotherapy treatment. As with glaucoma, cataracts can have a hereditary association, in which case it is important to have regular check-ups. Cataracts usually occur in both eyes, with one more severely affected. They are quite painless and develop slowly. They will not cause complete blindness. Nonetheless, they are disabling, since the main symptoms are blurred vision and disturbed colour vision.

MACULAR DEGENERATION

Degeneration may occur in the cells which make up the macula, the part of the retina responsible for central vision and sharp focus. The symptoms are usually blurred and distorted vision. If diagnosed early enough, it can be helped with laser treatment. Anti-oxidants may help the eyes on a cellular level as oxidation could be a primary cause of this condition.

IMPROVING YOUR EYESIGHT NATURALLY

Trayner pinhole glasses

These look like an ordinary pair of sunglasses but they contain numerous drilled holes of the diameter of a pin. Wearing them for just 15 minutes a day can exercise the eye muscles and help the eyes to focus better on their own. Trayner glasses can help with long- or short-sightedness; eye strain and headaches caused by prolonged close work on VDU screens. They can also relax tired eyes, build up your eyes' own flexibility, are suitable for both adults and children and can be used as a healthy form of sunglasses. You can wear them for watching TV, working at a VDU, during your normal everyday activities or relaxing outside. Trayner glasses are not meant as an alternative to conventional glasses but are intended purely to exercise the eyes. Whatever the problems they are beneficial. For further details apply to the address on page 218.

The Bates method

Dr William Horatio Bates devised this series of exercises to re-educate vision, relax strained eyes, retrain lazy muscles and generally improve eyesight. He was an opthalmologist who believed that many people wore glasses unnecessarily. Helped by a Bates Method teacher you will be taught a specific programme to suit your individual needs. It is a perfectly safe and non-invasive treatment, and it appears from anecdotal evidence that it can benefit people who suffer from long- or short-sightedness, astigmatism, lazy eyes and squints. It cannot reverse the effects of macular degeneration or cataracts. For further details contact the Bates Association (see page 218).

EYE NUTRITION

• Include plenty of anti-oxidant-rich foods in your diet, particularly those containing beta-carotene and anthocyanidins such as bilberry, grapeseed and pine bark.

• Vitamin A is helpful for many types of eye problem, including poor vision in dim light or at night.

• Vitamin B-complex is important for healthy eyes. A deficiency of vitamin B2 can lead to bloodshot, burning or gritty-feeling eyes, cataracts and sensitivity to bright lights.

• Vitamin C may preventat cataracts and glaucoma.

• Vitamin E helps to keep the blood vessels and retina healthy and is needed to prevent cataracts.

• Selenium can also prevent cataracts and slow the ageing of the eye.

• Zinc is required to release vitamin A from the liver for use by the eyes and is also needed in a high concentration by the retina to function properly.

emotional
factors

LIFE CHANGES
- Menopause
- Miscarriage
- Divorce
- Drug abuse
- Death
- Illness
- Stress

THERAPIES
- Relaxation
- Yoga
- Floatation
- Meditation
- Psychotherapy
- Hypnotherapy
- Autogenic training
- Body stress release
- Bach Flower Remedies

LIFE CHANGES

part one

Feelings are the building blocks of human knowledge. Now that we have discussed the various physiological changes which may occur as we grow older, we should also become aware of some of the emotional factors we could encounter.

First of all, how do we actually view the prospect of ageing? Society often seems to emphasize chronological age rather than focusing on mental age and quality of life. Chronological age and biological age resemble one another only in youth. To the very young ageing is something a long way away, but as we grow older it becomes associated with the clock in many people's minds.

Defining the period of life known as middle age is becoming less straightforward due to the fact that there has been a 70 per cent increase in life expectancy over the years. Our extended middle years should be perceived as our prime of life rather than the beginning of old age. Women seem to be judged more by their physical appearance than men, which often generates a fear of ageing. Grey hairs may depict advancing years in a woman, whereas in a man they are often seen as distinguished. Middle age should be a time of reassessment and a time to open the door to a new phase in maturity.

For instance, ask yourself whether in hindsight your life so far has been worth the effort, whether you have achieved your ambition or scope for self-expression and what hopes you have for the future. Your answers may help you to put your life into perspective and shape your future. You may feel that you have not had enough scope for self-expression – you were perhaps too busy bringing up a family. It is never too late to incorporate art, music, singing, drama and other interests into your life by joining a class or society specializing in one of these topics. We all have a hidden talent which very often goes completely undiscovered.

A woman may well have spent much of her earlier life bringing up a family and caring for her husband. Doing so much for others, she often neglects herself and may have even lost her own focus. According to Taoist philosophy, 'the wise woman waters her own garden first'. Through self-awareness

MAKE THE RIGHT CHOICE

Middle age is about choices: we can be destructive or constructive, negative or positive. At 50 plus we can either mourn our lost youth and fertility or we can see it as a time for second chances. Try to do the latter.

it is possible to enjoy a feeling of creativity, confidence, broader vision, better health and happiness.

Our way of life and circumstances certainly affect how quickly we age, but it is our psychological age – how old we *feel* we are – which plays such a significant role. If we expect to feel old at 50 or 60, then we will. However, individual circumstances can affect quality of life. For example, someone in a happy relationship who has a sense of humour and a healthy sex life, is positive about the future, can express her feelings easily, doesn't have too many financial burdens, enjoys her work or has satisfying hobbies and has a passion for something in life will grow old more slowly than someone who is lonely, unable to express her feelings or make changes, suffers from depression, dwells on the past, is unemployed or unhappy in her job and has no vision of the future.

There are various events that we may encounter along the path of life which will affect us emotionally. The main change which we women have in common is the menopause.

THE MENOPAUSE

The menopause is nature's verification that we are no longer able to bear children. Women consider it the last major change they will experience physiologically. However, as we discussed in chapter one, this doesn't have to be a change for the worse. For some women the menopause can create a sense of freedom. The factors listed opposite used to be thought of as part and parcel of the menopause – it was a woman's lot, to be suffered in silence. But nowadays things are different.

To begin with, women now feel able to discuss the subject openly. All the emotional and physical factors which accompany menopause can put a tremendous strain on a relationship. Sometimes it is difficult for a man to comprehend fully all the symptoms as he himself will never experience hormonal changes of such intensity during his life (though it is increasingly believed that men undergo a menopause of sorts, too). Communication is so important at this time, as couples who are able to converse openly about their feelings are less

REMEMBER
We should all aim to grow old gracefully and comfortably and die young mentally. Being young at heart is the maker of long life.

WORRIES AND FEARS
• The end of the child-bearing years.
• The ageing process will be accelerated by the menopause.
• Feelings of fading femininity.
• Sexual difficulties and loss of libido.
• Sleep problems.
• Mood swings.
• Weight gain due to a decline in the body's metabolism.

COPING ALONE

Not all women are in a marriage or relationship during their menopausal years, and although it is possible to consult a doctor with physiological problems, the emotional symptoms are not always addressed, leaving a woman feeling isolated and helpless. There are certain organizations (see page 219) specially for women in this situation; better still, try talking to someone in the same position who can relate to your feelings. Other ways of self-help are described later in this chapter.

WORRIES AND FEARS

• Discuss any anxieties with medical staff, who are becoming more aware of the importance of spending time with miscarriage sufferers, enabling them to communicate their emotions.
• The Miscarriage Association runs local support groups (see page 219).

likely to find the menopause a cause of strife. I have my own belief in HRT (Hormone Replacement Therapy, see page 71): in my view it should stand for Healthy Relationship Together.

During this time, other lifestyle changes may be taking place. If there are children, they may be growing up and experiencing adolescence. Important exams may be imminent, placing stress on the family, or the children may already be leaving home. This can often lead to the 'empty-nest syndrome', where a woman may feel she is no longer needed. She may actually miss the temperamental mood swings resulting from her children's raging hormones! Alternatively she might feel relief and value her new-found independence. Either way it can often come as a shock suddenly to find herself 'alone' again with a husband or partner, probably for the first time in around 18 years. Many couples fall into the habit of communicating with each other through their children, almost as if they are 'go-betweens'. When the nest becomes empty again, it is important to re-learn true communication with one another and to reawaken the love and friendship. Rekindle the flame by planning events together or taking up new interests.

There are many other lifestyle changes which may occur. Here are the main ones:

MISCARRIAGE

Miscarriage is a very distressing and often not fully understood event experienced by many women. It can trigger off a range of different emotions in both parents, including sadness, anger, feelings of helplessness, failure and a fear of future pregnancies.

One of the most traumatic aspects of miscarriage is that there is often no apparent explanation for its occurrence. It is vital to remember that miscarriages are relatively common and the fact that the pregnancy occurred means there is a strong likelihood of a healthy and successful pregnancy happening in the future.

Whether the reason for miscarriage was maternal or paternal will usually never be known but it is normally the woman who feels that she is responsible; there will no doubt be many 'if onlys' going round in her head. As with all upsetting events, women and men will cope and show their feelings differently. It is important for partners to communicate in order to understand each other's true feelings and be there to support one another. A man will often try to hide his grief, which can sometimes cause the woman to feel that he is not as upset as her, or that he is insensitive. In fact he may be concealing his feelings so as not to upset his partner further. Both partners may feel isolated even from family and friends as people often find it difficult to know what to say. For example, saying, 'You can always try again' does not really address the full extent of the couple's grief. No other child will completely replace a miscarried one. Unanswered questions will always remain, such as, 'Was it a boy or a girl?' The general advice is to accept the grief you experience as normal and realize that certain events – for instance, the date when the baby was due – is likely to rekindle sad feelings.

Lastly, bearing in mind that many miscarriages occur as a result of an abnormal foetus, it is a source of comfort that the body operates its own natural preventative mechanism. A *healthy* baby is, after all, what we all hope for.

BECOMING AN IN-LAW

The addition of new relationships to the family takes a little adjustment. All parents want the best for their offspring and naturally worry about them when they decide to set up home with a partner. They have to accept that a son's or daughter's visits may become less frequent as their time is occupied by their new way of life.

BECOMING A GRANDPARENT

Most people will liken becoming a grandparent to growing older and women do not always relish the idea of being called 'granny'. However, grandparenting can be a time of extreme pride and joy. You have after all acquired a new baby in the family without experiencing the pregnancy.

It is not uncommon for a grandmother to feel critical towards

BE POSITIVE
• Miscarriage is *not* uncommon.
• It does not preclude a healthy future pregnancy.
• Grieving is natural: do not push it away.

ENJOY BEING A GRANDPARENT
• Relish the joys of children without ultimate responsibility.
• Be prepared to help when help is asked for, but avoid unnecessary interference.

the nurturing of the grandchild. With the passage of time each generation has a different way of bringing up a child, but it is important to try to be supportive rather than intrusive.

Grandchildren can be extremely exhausting, so it is necessary to get plenty of rest before and after their visits. All in all they should bring happiness and give you the best of both worlds – the enjoyment without the responsibility.

WAYS OF COPING

• Remember that no two people cope with divorce in the same way.

• Give yourself time to mourn your loss rather than deny it.

• Don't be afraid to call on friends and family for support. Divorce is nothing to feel ashamed about.

• Contact a divorce or single-parent association (see page 219), or seek professional counselling. This is often beneficial for both divorcees and their children.

• Find someone with experience of a similar situation who will listen to you and not be judgmental. It is very important to offload rather than suppress emotions.

• Stress can damage your health, so make sure you look after yourself. Some approaches to controlling stress are discussed later in this chapter.

• Try to develop new interests or hobbies and take up a sport. This will stimulate the mind and the body and also help you to meet new friends.

DIVORCE

Whatever the cause or outcome, the break-up of a marriage or relationship can be an extremely stressful event. Marriage is an undertaking for which we hold great, though sometimes unrealistic, expectations. Feelings of anger, disbelief, failure, betrayal, resentment, inadequacy, sadness and worry are some of the many reactions we can experience. Alongside bereavement, divorce is a major stressor.

Yet divorce is not a solution to problems other than an unhappy marriage, and sometimes not the answer even for that. It cannot cure boredom, restlessness or general unhappiness and it is not a remedy for lack of self-worth, anxiety associated with middle age or any external problems. Wherever possible, it is better to solve the problems rather than using divorce as a way out of the situation. Sadly, now that divorce is so much easier, many people are rushing into it through errors of judgment.

Divorce demands many adjustments, emotional and circumstantial, which have to be considered fully before activating proceedings. A major change is moving away from or being left alone in the family home. If there are children involved, their feelings about the situation have to be taken into account. They may feel anxious, devastated, angry or betrayed and their reactions can vary from becoming completely introverted to rebelling totally. Children will very often blame themselves for their parents' divorce. Whatever the case, they should always be encouraged to express their feelings, a difficult task indeed for any parent who is already experiencing so much inner turmoil herself.

If the break-up or divorce is the result of an extra-marital affair in which one partner is being 'left' for another, this can cause a substantial loss of self-worth and esteem in the victim. Financial problems can be another stressful aspect. Division of property and assets, maintenance for children and decisions about pets all contribute to the strain.

DRUG ABUSE

Drug abuse is a problem of which many parents of teenage children need to be aware. In addition to smoking tobacco and drinking alcohol, which are socially acceptable to most people, there are many other substances, often referred to as recreational drugs, with strong mood-altering properties which can have dangerous effects on the mind and body. For adolescents who are still developing their sense of identity, the drug scene is an easy trap to fall into. They may try to deny feelings of insecurity in the escapism drugs offer. Parents should look out for warning signs such as mood swings and changes in the pupils of the eyes; they may find home-made cigarette stubs, needles, unusual substances or powders lying around; and they may notice that their child has a new circle of friends. For help and advice they can contact one of the organizations listed on pages 218 and 219.

Solvents

Solvents are usually inhaled as fumes from glues, cleaning fluids and lighter fuels and can cause giddiness, euphoria and loss of appetite. In large doses solvent abuse may lead to internal damage, asphyxiation and even heart failure.

Amphetamines

Amphetamines are stimulants usually swallowed as tablets but occasionally inhaled as powder or injected in solution form. The use of these stimulants can speed up the pulse and cause palpitations, dizziness, insomnia, paranoia and depression. Ecstasy, as recent tragic events have shown, is an amphetamine which can cause sudden death.

INDICATIONS OF DRUG ABUSE

- Home-made cigarette stubs.
- Needles or syringes.
- Unusual substances or powders.
- A new circle of friends.
- Anxiety or depression.

BEWARE

Recreational drugs are not always 100% pure. Many of the dangers lie in taking a substance whose contents are not known.

WARNING SIGNS

- Dilated or constricted pupils; bloodshot or swollen eyes.
- Nasal discharge.
- Change in behaviour.

WARNING SIGNS

- Dilated pupils and glare in the eyes.
- Hyperactivity.
- Bad breath; sometimes flushed skin.

WARNING SIGNS

- Weight loss.
- Nasal discharge.
- Change in personality.

Cocaine

Cocaine is also a stimulant, either inhaled or injected as cocaine hydrochloride powder or smoked as 'crack'. It induces a feeling of euphoria and self-confidence. This is because cocaine activates the receptor sites for the neurotransmitter dopamine and raises the levels in the brain, promoting a 'high'. It can also speed up the pulse, reduce appetite and cause feelings of anxiety and depression.

WARNING SIGNS

- Bloodshot eyes.
- Hunger.
- Mood swings.

Cannabis

Usually smoked or swallowed, cannabis comes in the form of the dried leaf, resin or oil of the plant. It can generate feelings of mild euphoria, sleepiness, talkativeness, hunger and dryness in the mouth. When smoked it can be damaging to the lungs as it is usually inhaled more deeply than normal cigarettes. Long-term use has been connected to impaired immune system response.

WARNING SIGNS

- Dilated pupils.
- Unpredictable behaviour.

LSD (Lyseric Acid Diethylamide)

LSD is swallowed in different forms and was very popular in the 1960s. It causes hallucinations, unbalanced sensations, paranoia and depression.

WARNING SIGNS

- Slurred speech.
- Constricted pupils.
- If heroin is injected, needlemarks, bruises and scars on the inside of the elbows; if inhaled, soreness around the nasal area.

Heroin

Derived from opium, heroin, like other opiates, copies the action of endorphins, the body's natural pain killers. Endorphin production is suppressed while someone is under the influence of heroin, but painful withdrawal symptoms can arise when heroin is stopped. These can include seizures, coma and sometimes death. For these reasons heroin withdrawal should be medically supervised.

WARNING SIGNS

- Bloodshot eyes.
- Mood swings.
- Unlike other substances, the smell of alcohol usually stays on the breath.

Alcohol

Despite being accepted socially in our culture, alcohol affects several of the body's neurotransmitters and reduces the functioning of the central nervous system. This can lead to the feeling of 'wobbly' legs and cause forgetfulness, giggling and drowsiness. In larger amounts it may cause slurred speech, memory loss and possibly coma or death. Combining alcohol with drugs can be very dangerous. Alcoholism is treatable so long as the problem is acknowledged. Drug therapy or psychotherapy is often advised or joining one of the alcohol associations (pages 218 and 219).

DEATH OF A LOVED ONE

Death is the one thing we all have in common. It is a universal experience but can have many different causes, such as old age, illness and accident. Bereavement is top of the list in stressful life events and can initiate various emotions. These include shock, disbelief, anger, guilt, regret, sadness and sometimes relief in cases of the terminally ill. Accompanying these emotional symptoms are many physical indications, such as loss of appetite, inability to sleep, palpitations, stomach upsets, skin conditions and chest pains.

Often the nature of death will have a marked bearing on how we actually cope with it. For example, the death of an elderly parent from illness after a long life will naturally cause grief and a great sense of loss. However, the adjustment will probably be easier than in the case of sudden death from an accident. There is likely to be more unresolved business after sudden death as there has been no time for goodbyes.

Death is often thought of as something which will not affect us, and until it happens to those close to us we never fully comprehend its real significance. It is at this time that we are suddenly reminded of our own mortality.

The death of a child is particularly hard to endure as we lose a part of ourselves and our future. In this situation feelings of guilt are very common and spouses often blame themselves, inevitably placing a tremendous strain on the relationship especially if one or both partners go into 'withdrawal'.

The death of a spouse, especially in old age, can create a total void in the remaining partner's life. Home suddenly becomes a very quiet, lonely place. Even friends experience embarrassment and inadequacy and often withdraw their

WAYS OF COPING

• Do talk about the deceased. Remember that 'To live in the hearts of those we love is not to die'.

• Recognize that there are no time limits on grief or pain; they are unfortunately the price we pay for loving someone.

• Learn to accept the fact that nothing will be the same again, but try to look optimistically to the future.

• Postpone any major decisions for at least six months; if made too hastily they could be regretted later on.

• Contact a bereavement counselling association (see page 219).

• Remember, you are lucky to have known love.

support. Upon the death of a spouse you suddenly, and involuntarily, revert to being single in a world which seems to be unusually full of couples.

REDUNDANCY AND UNEMPLOYMENT

Unfortunately, redundancy and unemployment seem to be a sign of our times. Both cause great stress. Emotions can range at this time from anger to boredom, depression and a sense of uselessness. To avoid feeling isolated it is important to have the support and encouragement of a partner or friends. While looking for work, try to make the most of the enforced free time by enrolling in an adult educational course. Many people have discovered a completely new and more rewarding career in this way. Join a gym or exercise class at a local leisure centre. The latter is more affordable as it is often government-subsidized. Without the routine of employment it is easy to lose motivation and become a couch potato, which in turn leads to apathy and depression.

RETIREMENT

Some people feel completely at a loose end when faced with retirement. It is a time when many adjustments need to be made. The best way to ensure an enjoyable retirement is to plan ahead and look forward to it. It does not have to signify inactivity, boredom and loneliness: by taking a positive attitude you should find it an extremely fulfilling, happy stage of your life. You will have the time available as never before to explore different interests. There may be a subject which you never had time to complete when young but which you could now take up again. Remember that learning is a never-ending process and should not cease the day you stop work. Naturally you will miss the daily or part-time routine to which you have been accustomed and also the company of work colleagues. However, giving up work does not have to mean relinquishing your friends.

Nowadays many people are choosing early retirement while others are opting for flexible retirement. If you want to

WAYS OF COPING

• Try to be positive and optimistic.

• Keep motivated by maintaining a daily routine.

• Read the papers regularly and keep up your social life; through meeting people you may learn of new openings.

• Take up courses (check to see if you are eligible for concessions) and exercise regularly. This will occupy you and stimulate your body and mind.

WAYS OF COPING

• Be positive. Cherish the freedom which accompanies retirement and look forward to a voyage of discovery.

• Ballroom dancing, exercise classes, bowls, yoga and golf are just a few ways of keeping fit and will introduce you to a new circle of friends.

• Check at your library for lists of courses available locally or consider a correspondence course. You may be eligible for concessionary rates.

• The Association of Retired Persons (see page 219) advises on pensions, insurance and health schemes.

• Some holiday companies cater for the over-60s, whether a theatre outing, a walking holiday or a coach tour.

continue working beyond the normal age for retirement and your employer is in agreement, then why not? Alternatively you may want to set up your own business, or work part-time as a fundraiser for your favourite charity.

ILLNESS

Coping with illness or disability can be extremely difficult for both sufferers and their families. A certain amount of adjustment is inevitable, but at the same time it is important not to give in to illness or impaired mobility. Emotionally coming to terms with an accident or illness is similar to coping with a bereavement, except in this case you are mourning the loss of movement, independence and general health.

Advancing technology has made possible many screening facilities for detecting health problems at an early stage, and the treatment available for conditions such as cataracts and replacements for joints has literally transformed the lives of many. Acquiring as much information as possible about the illness or condition will reduce the sufferer's anxiety and increase his/her understanding of the future prospects. It is also important that the sufferer is able to express emotions without feeling a burden to others, and that the doctor empathizes and communicates with the patient.

Caring for a sick relative can be emotionally depleting as it entails having to cope with both the nursing aspect and the moods of the sufferer. The carer may feel anger, guilt, resentment and perhaps loneliness. If as a carer or relative you feel unable to cope, contact the patient's doctor or a social worker. They will be able to arrange for counselling and care. There is also a course for carers that will teach you to give back to yourself what you are so busy giving to everyone else. It will help you identify your stresses and teach you techniques with which to overcome them. It will enable you to take action now before the effects of prolonged stress result in 'burn-out' or serious illness. It is ideal for nurses, doctors, social workers, counsellors, teachers and those in occupational health care. For details see page 219.

STRESS-ASSOCIATED SYMPTOMS

- Sweating.
- Dry mouth.
- Palpitations.
- Fainting.
- Headaches.
- Frequent urination.
- Digestive problems such as irritable bowel syndrome.

PHYSIOLOGICAL CHANGES

Stress has numerous affects on the body and mind. They include:

- High blood pressure.
- Allergies.
- Heart disease.
- Anorexia.
- Asthma.
- Hair loss.
- Cystitis.
- Eczema.
- Ulcers.
- Headaches and migraine.
- Epilepsy.
- Insomnia.
- Indigestion.
- Menstrual problems.
- Weight loss or weight gain.
- Addictions such as alcoholism and drug dependency.

STRESS

Stress places an excessive strain on the mind and body, but despite its poor reputation it is one of the body's best defence systems. In times of danger our adrenal glands release adrenaline, making us more alert and increasing our strength.

None of us is immune to stress; indeed, a certain amount of stress is good for us as it keeps us motivated and active and can boost performance. Whether we are speaking in public, competing in a sports event, sitting an exam or appearing on stage, it can add an edge to the event. Too little stress may mean that we lack the drive to achieve our aims.

However, too much stress can in the long term be very destructive to health. It is important to identify the cause of stress once you have recognized the signs and symptoms and remember that it is not always unpleasant events which activate stress. For example, marriage, childbirth and Christmas can all be happy occasions, but they can also be stressful.

The level of stress experienced depends largely on the way it is perceived and interpreted. There are usually three phases in our response to stress: the event itself, our inner assessment of it, and our body's reaction to it. It is the second phase which is the vital connection to the end result: in other words, our mental judgement of a situation can have a profound effect on our body's response.

A certain amount of stress is inevitable in the case of life events such as those described earlier in this chapter. It is the needless stress, such as arguing unnecessarily, which will cause long-term problems. Overwork often causes stress to the point where illness is the end result. Long-term pain can lead to a feeling of helplessness. It is important not to become a victim of the type of stress over which you have control.

DEPRESSION

Each year an increasing number of people consults their doctors for depression. It is a word used to describe a wide spectrum of moods which, perhaps inevitably, are often misunderstood. Sometimes when people say they are feeling depressed, all they really mean is that they are fed up, sad or feeling a bit under the weather.

Nowadays experts tend to categorize depression in terms of degree. For instance, *mild* depression, which may occur after an upset, leaves you feeling low but still able to cope with everyday life; *moderate* depression reduces normal functioning; and *severe* depression is a chronic condition which can often prevent the sufferer from thinking clearly, being able to get out of bed and going to work.

There is usually an obvious cause for depression such as marital break-up, death of someone close, financial or legal problems or unemployment. The common emotions associated with these, such as feelings of failure, betrayal and disappointment, can all create depression. Some people are better able to cope with stress and anxiety, whereas others are more easily upset and more prone to depression depending on their personality and circumstances.

Sometimes depression will not lift. Months pass by without any relief, to the extent where it eventually becomes an illness. This is when help should be sought. Before embarking on treatment it is important to realize that there is nothing to feel ashamed of. Depression is extremely common and highly treatable, and remember – you are not alone. An untreated depression can deepen or it may subside, but nine times out of ten it is likely to recur.

According to Kimberley Yonkers, MD, assistant professor of psychiatry and gynaecology at the University of Texas South Western Medical Center in Dallas, 'There's a theory that depression revolves around anger, in that women in general tend to suppress their anger, turn it inwards and, as a result get depressed. Men on the other hand outwardly express their anger and rage by getting aggressive.' Women, however, are more inclined to seek guidance, particularly if they are not receiving much support at home. They are generally more able to uncover their emotions to a therapist than men are.

Sadly, depression is frequently overlooked or neglected and many cases are believed to go unrecognized and untreated.

SYMPTOMS OF DEPRESSION
- **Feelings of isolation.**
- **Feelings of despair.**
- **Lack of self-worth.**
- **Tearfulness.**
- **Inability to concentrate.**
- **General loss of interest in life.**

WAYS OF COPING
- **Talk to someone who will listen.**
- **Try writing your negative thoughts down on paper.**
- **Do not turn to drugs or alcohol for comfort: in the long run they will only exacerbate the problem.**
- **Take up exercise (see chapter four) – it increases brain activity and releases certain neurotransmitters (chemical messenger substances) which help to uplift the mood.**
- **Join a support group (see page 219).**
- **Indulge in any of the therapies listed in chapter three or one of the procedures for controlling stress and depression described in this chapter.**

Don't suffer in silence: depression does not have to destroy your life so long as you seek help. There are many ways of coping and various effective treatments available.

Cognitive therapy

Cognitive therapy is often used successfully in the treatment of depression. It helps sufferers to alter their present way of thinking by destroying negative thinking and replacing it with a more realistic and optimistic outlook. Cognitive therapists can teach techniques for managing stress and anxiety and will also encourage their patients to take up certain activities in order to create a sense of achievement. Cognitive therapy works very well for anxiety, bereavement and post-traumatic stress in addition to depression.

WAYS OF COPING

• Go outside more, even if it isn't sunny. The fresh air will do you good.

• Keep fit to balance your hormones.

• Try to wear brighter-coloured clothes.

• Ask your doctor about the possibility of melatonin supplements.

• Try phototherapy. This involves exposing the eyes to very bright light, which stimulates the hormonal system, in particular the pineal gland. It is available as a light box which shines on you while you are watching television or working at a desk. You do not have to look directly into the light. Using the light box for half an hour a day will revive the pineal gland and lift the associated depression.

• Contact the the SAD Association for more information (see page 219).

SEASONAL AFFECTIVE DISORDER

Another form of depression experienced by many people, especially during the winter months, is seasonal affective disorder (SAD). It occurs as a result of lack of good-quality light and an underactive pineal gland.

The pineal gland, which is the size of a pea and situated deep within the brain, regulates the secretion of the hormone melatonin which controls our sleep-wake cycle. Its association with light is very significant as there is an intimate relationship between light exposure and melatonin levels. In some people the dim light of winter causes abnormal rhythms in the production of melatonin which accordingly confuse the setting of their body clock. The pineal gland then has to secrete more melatonin, which can consequently make us feel sleepy and lethargic. In turn, the hypothalamus (the brain's control centre) decreases its production of serotonin, a neurotransmitter which keeps us feeling happy and relaxed.

Sufferers of SAD are often naturally deficient in serotonin and this, combined with the low levels of available light during the winter months, can cause a variety of symptoms such as oversleeping, feeling listless, craving starchy or sugary foods, boredom and loss of libido.

THERAPIES

It is widely acknowledged that the wellbeing of our bodies is linked to our emotional state. In part one, we discussed possible emotional reactions to major changes in our lives, and reviewed how these can adversely affect our health. The importance of seeking help, being prepared to undertake therapies and of communication with friends and family cannot be emphasized enough. There *is* usually a way out of our troubles. Some of the following therapies and remedies are cheap and easy to do at home, others require professional help or equipment.

part two

The following ways to help reduce stress and depression and promote relaxation are just a few of the many available.

Relaxation

Relaxation is a necessity for good physical and mental health, and not just something to be experienced once a year while on holiday. Regular relaxation should be part of daily life. Although many people feel that watching television or reading is a way of relaxing, the brain and the eyes are in fact still very active.

Relaxation does not need any equipment; it costs nothing except time and motivation. It is extremely beneficial in cases of stress, depression, muscular tension, headaches, PMT, high blood pressure, insomnia and many other conditions.

RELAXATION THROUGH BREATHING

An important part of relaxation involves centring on the way we breathe. There is a yogic saying: 'Breath is life'. When feeling anxious, we tend to take shallow breaths from the upper chest. This increases anxiety and reduces energy although it is fine during exercise as it delivers a quick boost of oxygen to the system. For relaxation, correct breathing from the diaphragm not only oxygenates the body more, but also prevents a build-up of carbon dioxide in the lungs, thereby enhancing health.

BENEFITS

Relaxation can help:

• Maintain good physical and mental health.

• Reduce the harmful effects of stress.

• Relieve muscular tension and headaches.

• Reduce blood pressure.

• Aid restful sleep.

• Alleviate the symptoms of PMT.

• Keep oxygen levels at an optimum.

Targeted breathing exercises

Find a quiet, well-ventilated area where you will be able to relax undisturbed.

❶ Lie on your back with your eyes closed. You may find it helpful to place an object such as a book on your abdomen in order to focus your mind on its movement with the breathing. Keeping your mouth closed, breathe in deeply through your nose but from the diaphragm, focusing your attention on your abdomen which should rise as you inhale.

❷ Hold the breath without tensing for about five seconds and then breathe out slowly through your mouth.

❸ Gradually increase the number of seconds for inhaling and exhaling so that your breathing becomes regular, rhythmic and balanced.

The exercise illustrated below works just as well sitting at your desk, or standing. Practise it in any spare moment you have.

❶ Kneel, with your shoulders in line with the hips, and straighten your back. Lengthen the neck; do not tense it.

❷ Breathe in slowly through the nose, at the same time trying to imagine the stomach muscles being pulled through to the spine.

❸ Hold the breath for about five seconds, then slowly release.

If you practise breathing for relaxation for about ten minutes each day, you will soon be able to do it travelling on buses and trains or even in traffic jams. In the last instance be sure to keep your eyes open, though!

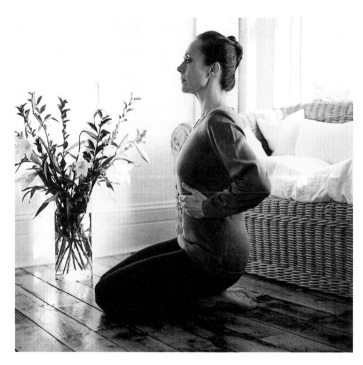

RELAX YOUR MIND

Provided all your muscles are relaxed and your focus is on your breathing, there will be no need to try to relax your mind. Some people like to visualize light blue as a cleansing colour as they inhale and a darker colour such as brown for exhaling the unclean.

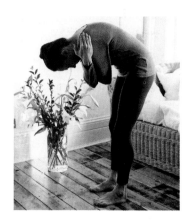

This exercise makes you aware how deeply you breathe and releases tension from the lower back.

❶ Stand upright with your feet in line with your shoulders and knees slightly bent.

❷ With your shoulders and arms relaxed, hug yourself gently, then bend forward from the waist.

❸ Breathe in and out slowly for a few minutes. This will open out the upper back, stretching the length of the spine and opening out the ribs.

PROGRESSIVE MUSCULAR RELAXATION

In the body there are numerous skeletal muscles which naturally contract when we are feeling stressed, creating muscular tension. Progressive muscular relaxation is aimed at loosening the effects of stress by relaxing the muscle groups individually. By systematically flexing and unleashing the muscles, this method of relaxation, if practised regularly, will promote a healthier mind and body.

The idea is to work progressively through the body area by area. It is best to wear loose clothing and lie on your back either on the floor or a bed. Starting with your toes, work all the way up the legs through the calves, knees and thighs to the buttocks, stomach, back, shoulders, neck, fingers, arms and every facial muscle. First clench the muscles in the chosen area as hard as possible, emphasizing the tension in that area. Hold for about five to ten seconds (this can gradually be increased) and then completely relax the same muscles.

In all, this should take around ten to 15 minutes. It will bring about awareness of the areas in which you hold the most tension, and when combined with the breathing exercises, will promote deep relaxation.

❶ To relax and lengthen the spine, kneel on the floor, then bend forward so that your forehead touches the floor. Keep your arms in line with your legs.

❷ Try to push your bottom towards the floor, to get more of a stretch (this may be easier with a small cushion placed underneath).

❸ Stay in this position for as long as you feel comfortable, about 2–3 minutes.

RELAXATION OF THE SPINE

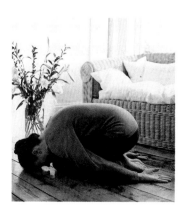

Yoga

BENEFITS

Yoga, a joining of mind and body, has existed for thousands of years. It can greatly enhance the health of mind and body and lead to a peaceful inner awareness by:

• Reducing tension, depression fatigue, anger and anxiety.

• Helping conditions such as back pain, headache, high blood pressure, PMT and digestive problems.

• Benefiting anyone leading a sedentary lifestyle.

• Increasing flexibility, vitality and concentration levels.

BEWARE

• If you are taking any medication or have any physical problems or injuries, it is best to consult your doctor before learning yoga.

• Start by taking lessons with a qualified teacher. Once you have mastered the techniques you will be able to practise at home.

• Wear loose clothing and avoid sessions directly after a meal.

Originating in India about 1500 years ago, yoga literally translated from Sanskrit means union. The ancient yogis perceived the physical body as a vehicle with the mind as its driver and the soul as man's true existence. Yoga is a method of balancing these three forces.

One of the great masters of yoga, Swami Vishnu Devananda, compares the human body to a car. It needs lubrication, a cooling system, an electric current, fuel and a sensible driver behind the wheel for it to run properly. He developed five principles to fulfill these functions.

◆ The asanas (positions) *lubricate* the body, keep the muscles and joints running smoothly, tone all the internal organs and increase circulation without creating any fatigue.

◆ The body is *cooled* by complete relaxation.

◆ Pranayama (yogic breathing) increases prana, *electric current*.

◆ *Fuel* is provided by the food and water we consume together with the air we breathe.

◆ Lastly there is meditation, the *driver* which stills the mind and transcends the body – the physical vehicle.

There are many different branches of yoga but hatha is the most practised form in the west. The word hatha comes from the Sanskrit meaning sun and moon and implies the union of opposites. It works on the physical aspects of body control.

It is not necessary to have any particular spiritual beliefs to practise yoga. Whatever your age, it can enhance your lifestyle and benefit health. There is no special equipment needed other than a yoga mat, available from the Sivananda Yoga Vedanta Centre (see page 219) or you may like to buy a lotus chair, which is ideal for yoga, meditation and expectant mothers. Alternatively you could use a folded towel to lie on.

Yoga's health-giving and rejuvenating properties are available to all. It can help elderly people to retain their mobility – they often find that it relieves arthritis and poor circulation. Some of the asanas can be beneficial for pregnant women, alleviating

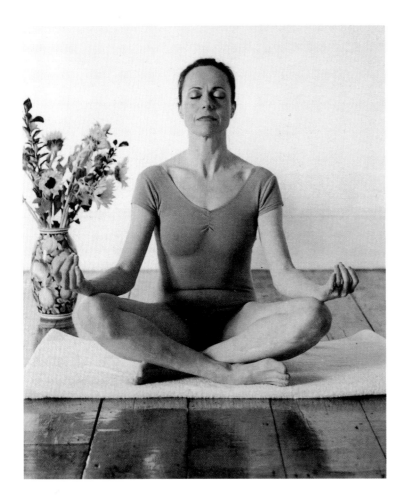

THE HALF LOTUS

The half lotus (or easy sitting position) is much safer for beginners. Try this before progressing to the full lotus.

Sit on the floor, keeping your back straight, and pull yourself up out of the hips. Take care not to hunch the shoulders. Rest the back of your hands on your knees and join the tips of thumb and index finger.

problems such as backache, promoting the health of the unborn child and sometimes helping shorten labour. Yoga also benefits those practising sport as it helps to build and balance muscular strength, thereby lessening the chance of injury.

If yoga is combined with regular relaxation and meditation, the benefits to health are immeasurable. The body's flexibility will improve and vitality will increase from the relaxation and breathing techniques through the raised level of oxygen to the brain, and concentration will be heightened through meditation.

On the following pages the salute to the sun should be performed in the order shown, following the circle of the sun.

SUN SALUTATION

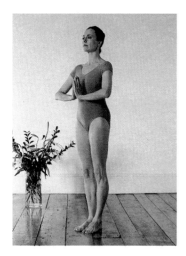

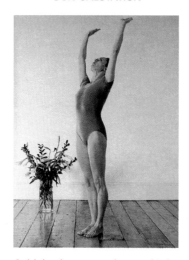

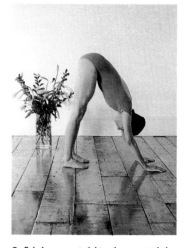

1 Stand up straight with your feet together and arms relaxed by your sides. Breathe deeply and, as you bring your palms together, exhale. Keeping your head relaxed, look straight ahead.

2 Inhale, raise your arms above your head and arch gently backwards. Keep your knees and elbows straight and make sure your palms are facing upwards. Reach back with your head.

3 Exhale and bend forwards without bending your knees. Aim to place your palms flat on the floor beside your feet; otherwise reach down as far as you can. Tuck your head in against the knees.

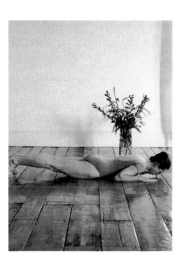

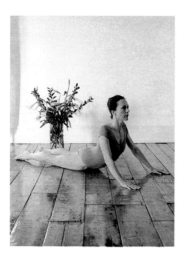

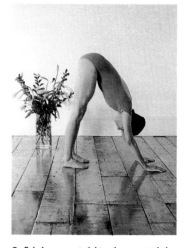

7 Inhaling, shift your body forward and take your weight on the hands. Bring the chest and forehead to the floor (as shown). Then, exhaling, push your hips up. Ideally the knees should be resting on the floor.

8 Inhale and, without moving the hands, arch the chest back and stretch your head up as far as is comfortable. This is known as the cobra pose.

9 Exhale as you straighten the arms, tuck the toes under and push up the hips. Keep your hands and feet flat on the floor, your legs and back straight and drop the head directly between the arms.

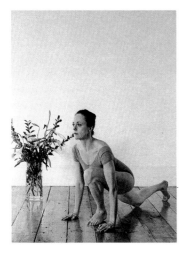

4 Keeping your hands in the same position, inhale and push your right leg back as far as possible. Drop the right knee to the floor. Look up and push the pelvis forward.

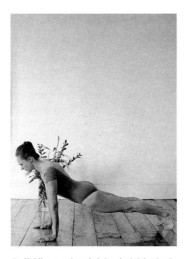

5 Holding your breath, bring the left leg back so that it aligns with the right, with the toes pointing forwards. Keep your neck in a straight line with the spine. Do not arch the back or lift or drop the hips.

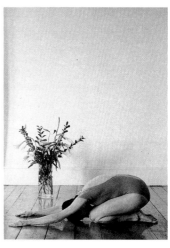

6 Exhale and move your body backwards. Keep your hands in the same position until you are resting back on your heels and your forehead touches the floor.

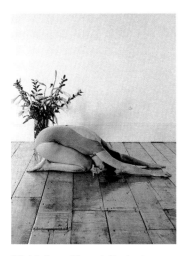

10 Inhaling and then exhaling, bend your knees, rest back on your heels and lightly place your forehead on the floor. Your arms should stay in front of you, with the palms flat on the floor.

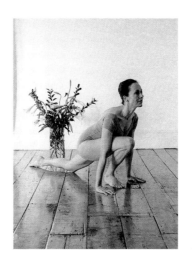

11 Keeping your hands in the same position, inhale, bring your right knee up between your hands and push your left leg back. Drop the left knee to the floor, look up and push the pelvis forward.

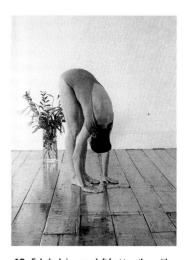

12 Exhale, bring your left foot together with your right and repeat as for step 3. Finally, inhale, uncurl the spine gradually, leaving the head to come up last. Repeat the salute, starting at position 1 if you wish to.

Floatation

BENEFITS

These include:

• Anxiety.

• Insomnia.

• Muscular tension.

• For further details and the address of your nearest floatation centre contact the Floatation Tank Association (see page 219).

Unlikely though it may sound, flotation can help to relieve stress and stress-related problems by promoting deep relaxation. Anyone can float, whether they are able to swim or not. The water in a floatation cabin or tank is only 25cm/10in deep and, because of the mixture of Epsom and other mineral salts in the water, your body is totally supported so that you cannot help floating.

The temperature of the water is controlled at 34.2°C/93.56°F, which is normal skin temperature. The salts in the water ensure that your skin will not become crinkly!

A floatation session normally lasts for an hour, although some people even enjoy overnight sessions! You float on your back, resting your head on an air pillow if you choose. It is advisable to wear the ear plugs which are always provided to prevent water from entering the ears.

Soft gentle music can be played through underwater speakers or, if you wish, you can relax in a completely soundless environment. You can also opt for a dim light, which you can control, or complete darkness. It is necessary to shower before and after a session to wash off the salts on the skin. The water is filtered after every session, so it is completely hygienic.

Floatation provides the perfect opportunity to unwind. Without normal outside sensations, such as light and sound, the brain tends to turn inwards, allowing a feeling of inner awareness. Each person seems to experience a different sensation when floating. Many people have reported an increased level of concentration, inspiration, accelerated learning abilities and relief of muscle and joint pain due to the wonderful feeling of weightlessness.

A floatation tank is an ideal place to meditate. Some people who are undergoing psychotherapy or hypnotherapy (see pages 104 and 105) take the opportunity to listen to their own live or pre-recorded therapy tapes.

Meditation

In India and other parts of Asia meditation (finding an inner peace) has been practised for thousands of years as a means of achieving spiritual awareness. In our stressful lives today such moments of calm are very rare and should be treasured.

Becoming a master of your mind rather than servant to it, you will discover the peace and enlightenment which lie within. During meditation, the hypothalamus (the brain's control centre for emotions as well as certain physical functions) actually expands, leading to a feeling of peace and increased creativity.

Meditation can be practised in a group or on your own. If meditating on your own, choose somewhere with a quiet atmosphere where you will be undisturbed. It is best to sit either on the floor cross-legged and with your arms resting on your knees, or in a chair with your back well supported. Begin by relaxing your breathing so that it becomes slower, deeper and rhythmic. Relax your mind but do not force it to concentrate; just let your thoughts drift away. Focusing the eyes on the flame of a candle can be relaxing; alternatively close your eyes and focus your mind on something within such as the heart chakra (centre). Blocking off the senses is another helpful way of reaching a higher level of concentration. You can do this by covering your ears with your thumbs, your eyes with your index fingers, your nostrils with your middle fingers (releasing them to breathe in) and your lips with your fourth and fifth fingers.

Playing soothing music or a meditation or relaxation tape can help you attain a meditative state. Begin with ten-minute sessions and gradually increase the time as and when you feel it is necessary.

Practised on a regular basis, meditation should improve your ability to cope mentally and physically with stress and everyday problems such as insomnia, high blood pressure and most stress-induced conditions.

BENEFITS

Meditation, the medicine of the mind, is a way of centralizing the thoughts and calming the body. By focusing the mind on one central point you are more able to achieve self-awareness.

• Provides a moment of peace in a busy, frantic day.

• Increases creativity.

• Improves mental capacity and focuses the mind.

• Reduces the effects of stress.

• Helps overcome insomnia.

• Brings a higher level of spiritual awareness.

Psychotherapy

BENEFITS

Psychotherapy is beneficial in treating cases of:

• Insomnia.

• Compulsive behaviour.

• Phobias.

• Neuroses.

• Stress.

• Depression.

BEWARE

Make sure that your therapist is registered with a professional organization such as:

• The British Association for Counselling.

• The UK Council for Psychotherapy.

• The British Confederation of Psychotherapists.

• The British Psychological Society.

• The National Council of Psychotherapists and Hypnotherapy.

• The National Register of Hypnotherapists and Psychotherapists (see page 000 for all details).

Deriving from the Greek *psyche,* meaning mind, and *therapeutikos,* meaning to treat or attend to, psychotherapy is traditionally accepted as arising from the work of Sigmund Freud (1856–1939). He was one of the first to move away from the belief that memory was a fairly simple process. Human beings were hitherto supposed to be rational (if wilful) creatures who were aware of what they were doing. Freud unearthed a discrepancy between the unconscious mind and the conscious mind. He concluded that some of our behaviour is controlled by stimuli of which we are completely unaware but may be triggered by a storehouse of memories not normally accessible to the human mind.

Psychotherapists are *not* usually medically trained and so will not prescribe drugs and treatments such as shock therapy. Instead they are trained to help people with problems too deep to be solved by normal means or counselling.

Psychotherapy sometimes takes the client back to childhood, a time when pain and fears have been suppressed to the extent that by adulthood they have become deeply buried. This often gives rise to feelings of low self-worth. The therapist treats the 'whole person', enabling the client to understand the many diverse areas of his/her mind. This method helps the client to break free from restrictive routine behaviour and attain a clearer picture of his/her hopes and desires. It is essential that a deep and trusting relationship is formed between therapist and client and that there is a complete commitment to the therapy. This will heighten the client's own healing powers.

It is not necessary to be experiencing a crisis to benefit from psychotherapy; it can also help to enrich relationships and improve the quality of life. Counsellors and psychotherapists often work alongside the Health Service and voluntary organizations although there is often a waiting list for treatment. If you feel psychotherapy might help you, ask your doctor for a referral.

Hypnotherapy

As hypnotherapy is an excellent way of reaching the unconscious mind, it can complement psychotherapy. It works at a deeper level of consciousness by seeking to create mental and physical changes which will in turn heal physical illness. With the aid of subconscious learning, clients can gain an insight into past difficulties and understand how they inform present problems. The benefits of hypnotherapy are completely 'holistic' because it treats the whole person. With time clients gain self-confidence by reliving and accepting past events and so become able to look forward positively to the future.

BENEFITS

Hypnotherapy reaches the unconscious mind and so can complement psychotherapy. It can:
• Improve physical health.
• Reveal the deep-rooted sources of emotional problems.
• Increase self-confidence.
• Help foster an optimistic outlook.

Autogenic training

Autogenic training was developed in the late 1920s by German neurologist Dr Johannes Schultz. Realizing the benefits of complete relaxation induced by hypnosis, he set out to create a method of relaxation which did not require actual hypnosis. He devised a set of exercises which became so successful that the training was taken up in Europe, North America and Japan.

AT teaches clients to use the exercises for themselves. The training can be continued on an individual basis or in small groups. The series of simple mental exercises assist the body's self-regulatory actions. Before starting AT, the client completes a health questionnaire to determine the appropriate course.

AT is unusual among other relaxation techniques in that it aims to rebalance the brain's inherent functions and the activities of its right and left hemispheres. This encourages the release of repressed feelings of anger, bitterness, fear and sadness. It teaches you to let go, to stop constantly striving for results and encourages you to become a more passive observer. This leads to a stronger immune system, greater inner healing, emotional balance and a marked increase in creativity.

BENEFITS

Physiological disorders such as:
• High blood pressure.
• Asthma.
• IBS.
• Migraine.
• Bladder problems.
• Arthritis.
• Skin complaints.
• Immune system problems such as ME and Aids.

Psychological conditions such as:
• Anxiety.
• Grief.
• Stress.
• Sleep disturbances.
• Stammering.
• Phobias.
• Alcohol dependence.

Body stress release

BENEFITS

Body stress release is not yet widely practised but is proven effective in:
• Locating points where tension is stored and releasing that stored tension.
• Reducing physical stress in elderly people from falls and the stressful effects of childbirth on mother and child.
• Healing physical injuries.
• Counteracting the harmful effects of chemical pollution.

Body stress release is a technique devised by Ewald and Gail Meggersee in South Africa eleven years ago. He is an osteopath and she is a qualified chiropractitioner. Although successful in these therapies, they both became dissatisfied with their limitations in treating the effects of certain types of stress on the body. Body stress release is now very popular in South Africa, but still relatively unknown in the UK.

What causes body stress?

Body stress can have emotional or physical causes. We may suffer various emotional and mental stress factors, such as fear of the future, financial worries and breakdown in family relationships. Both ongoing forms of mental strain, such as anxiety, and sudden emotions, such as anger or shock, can manifest themselves as body stress.

Mechanical stress occurs as a result of various jerks, bumps and falls which to a certain extent the body is able to withstand, but sometimes its limit of adaptability is exceeded. We are also subject to chemical stress factors from sources such as pollutants in the air, insecticides, food additives and preservatives. These are consumed, inhaled or absorbed through skin contact.

The body is designed to be self-healing and is capable of repairing wounds and fractures, counteracting harmful chemicals and adapting to sudden changes in temperature. When the point of stress overload is reached, however, the individual's ability to adapt diminishes. Instead of stress being released from the body it is then stored as body stress.

Stress can lock memory into the cells and becomes manifest in tension, tiredness and lack of energy and enthusiasm. As a result headaches, backache and digestive problems can occur. While the stress and tension remain stored in the body, the normal tone of the body becomes disturbed, causing a reduction in its general efficiency. It then becomes less and less able to deal with further daily stresses until eventually the general state of health diminishes. The person experiencing this may simply come to accept as normal the sense of feeling less than 100 per cent well.

The body stress release technique

With the person fully clothed and lying down, the practitioner will locate the exact sites of the body stress by applying light pressure to various points on the body and observing the response. In this way the body acts as a biofeedback mechanism, supplying the necessary information.

To encourage the body to release its stored tension, the practitioner then applies a stimulus by means of light but definite pressure on the relevant areas. If there is long-term stress stored in the body, its release is likely to take longer.

The body stress release technique is not a diagnosis or treatment of a specific condition or disease. It is concerned only with locating and releasing stored tension which in turn will promote optimum health.

Two to three sessions on a weekly basis are usually recommended, although deeper structural problems such as frozen shoulder or sciatica may need more treatments. The first session releases the basic stress, the second session has a more healing effect and the third should see the body begin to settle down more. As a follow up the therapist may suggest another treatment after a month. Light massage, aromatherapy and gentle yoga work very well alongside body stress release.

Who can benefit?

Anyone can benefit from the treatment, from infants to the elderly, whether sick or healthy. A baby may suffer body stress after a difficult birth, as will the mother. Elderly people who are prone to falls could suffer not only from physical stress but also from fear of further falls.

Body stress release, together with minimizing stress overload, allows individuals the opportunity of expressing their highest potential.

Bach Flower Remedies

BENEFITS

Dr Bach devised a structure of seven major groups, into which people could be categorized:

• Fear.

• Uncertainty.

• Insufficient interest in present circumstances.

• Loneliness.

• Oversensitivity to influences and ideas.

• Despondency or despair.

• Overcare for the welfare of others.

The Bach Flower Remedies are a collection of preparations produced from wild flowers and plants by Dr Edward Bach. A Harley Street consultant, bacteriologist and homeopath, in 1930 he relinquished his lucrative practice in London to expand his knowledge of the plant world. His belief was that 'a healthy mind ensures a healthy body' and that inner conflict is the cause of most illnesses. With this in mind, he developed 38 remedies which constitute a complete system of healing. Each plant was chosen to work on a particular emotional state, and the collection *in toto* accommodates every negative feeling.

Dr Bach discovered the first remedies Impatiens and Mimulus in Wales. He then found a further 17 before moving to Mount Vernon, a beautiful country house near Oxford. There he completed his collection with a further 19 remedies taken from plants growing in the area. He died in 1936, but Mount Vernon remains the Bach Centre, where the remedies are prepared.

Dr Bach's intuition and his sensitivity to people's emotions were highly developed. He could tell instinctively what mental state a plant related to, and in many cases suffered greatly from an emotion until he found the flower that would help him.

BEWARE

• Bach flower remedies will support other treatments and can be taken alongside orthodox medicine but they do not replace medical attention. It is always advisable to seek medical advice when necessary.

HOW TO TAKE THE REMEDIES

Take two drops of your chosen remedy or remedies in a glass of mineral water or fruit juice. Take the doses four times daily: first thing in the morning, last thing at night and twice in between. In an emergency they can be dropped directly on to the tongue, but this is an expensive way of taking them.

The most effective method is to make up a treatment bottle. Put two drops from each remedy into a 30ml/1fl oz bottle and fill up with natural spring water (non-carbonated). Take four drops in a teaspoon of water as often as needed, but at least four times a day and especially first and last thing daily. Hold the dose in the mouth for a few moments before swallowing. The remedies can also be added to a bath or to massage oil.

The length of treatment will depend on your personal reaction to the remedies as well as on how long you have suffered from the condition and how severe it is. Sometimes there will be no change for the first two weeks, but it is important to persevere. Stop taking the remedies when you feel that you no longer have the need for them. If you prefer, you can consult a fully qualified therapist specializing in Bach Flower Remedies (see page 219 for where to obtain details of therapists in your area).

Whatever is inhibiting you in life, the Bach Flower Remedies will help your emotional state and control negative feelings before, during and after certain events in your life. They act like an invisible hand – unseen and unheard – but our real healing is within us. All it needs is reawakening. As Dr Bach himself said, 'There is no true healing unless there is a change in outlook, peace of mind and inner happiness.'

RESCUE REMEDY

The Bach Rescue Remedy, a unique combination of five of the Flower Remedies, is for use in emergencies. Four drops from the stock bottle should be taken in water; alternatively, tablets are available from Nelson's Pharmacy, (see page 219). The Rescue Remedy is composed as follows:

- Star of Bethlehem – for shock.
- Rock Rose – for great fear and terror.
- Impatiens – for mental agitation.
- Cherry Plum – for fear of the mind giving way.
- Clematis – for dreaminess or distant feelings.

BENEFICIARIES

Animals as well as humans can benefit from the remedies, particularly the Rescue Remedy. For small animals just add four drops to their drinking water or milk; for larger creatures add ten drops to a bucket of water. Plants also thrive when watered with the addition of Rescue Remedy.

Also available is the Bach Rescue Cream which can be beneficial for various skin complaints and burns. It does not contain lanolin.

THE RESCUE REMEDY

This has been carefully prepared to create an all-round combination which helps in a crisis or stressful everyday situations such as:

- Going to the dentist.
- Taking an exam.
- Wedding-day nerves.
- Working to a tight deadline.
- Arriving late for an important meeting.
- Going for a job interview.
- Moving house.
- Coping with bereavement.
- Facing redundancy.
- Jangled nerves after an argument.
- Stage fright.
- Receiving bad news.

THE EMOTIONS AND THEIR RELEVANT REMEDIES

When choosing a remedy or remedies, it is important that you first recognize your emotion. This can be difficult as negative emotions are hard to confess, but once you have acknowledged and faced up to them they are easy to treat.

FEAR

Fear of known things – possibly fear of food in cases of anorexia, shyness, timidity, self-consciousness.
Remedy: **Mimulus**

Fears and worries of unknown origin – apprehension.
Remedy: **Aspen**

Fear of the mind giving way – uncontrolled thoughts, feeling out of control or suicidal, experiencing violent impulses.
Remedy: **Cherry Plum**

Fear or overconcern for others – not worrying about oneself but worrying incessantly about the well-being of loved ones.
Remedy: **Red Chestnut**

Terror – extreme panic attacks, great fear: for example, of an accident or sudden illness.
Remedy: **Rock Rose**

UNCERTAINTY

Lethargy and procrastination – mental fatigue, that 'Monday morning' feeling, a feeling that something that was once a pleasure now seems a chore.
Remedy: **Hornbeam**

Hopelessness and despair – pessimism, defeatism, loss of the will to fight in very ill people, affliction with SAD.
Remedy: **Gorse** (Gorse is known as 'sunshine in a bottle')

Uncertainty and indecision – mood swings, inner conflict, a need to bring thoughts into focus, travel sickness.
Remedy: **Scleranthus**

Discouragement and despondency – doubt, discouragement due to setbacks or other known causes in life.
Remedy: **Gentian**

Uncertainty as to the correct path in life – sensation of being at a crossroads in life, feeling a need to bring out a special talent in oneself which has been suppressed or a need to fulfil new ideas, difficulty in making any sort of commitment.
Remedy: **Wild Oat**

Seeking confirmation in others – needing other people's opinions because of a lack of confidence in and doubt in one's own judgement and so being unable to act on one's own intuition.
Remedy: **Cerato**

INSUFFICIENT INTEREST IN PRESENT CIRCUMSTANCES

Lack of energy – exhaustion, physical and mental, weakness after illness.
Remedy: **Olive**

Living in the past – nostalgia, inability to bring oneself into the present.
Remedy: **Honeysuckle**

Dreaminess, lack of interest in the present – absent-mindedness, daydreaming to escape from life or reality.
Remedy: **Clematis**

Deep gloom with no origin – depression for an unknown reason, affliction with SAD.
Remedy: **Mustard**

Failure to learn from past mistakes – nothing seems to sink in, may apply to some children, perhaps with learning disabilities.
Remedy: **Chestnut Bud**

Resignation and apathy – negativity, resignation to the fact that one will never get better.
Remedy: **Wild Rose**

Unwanted thoughts – mental arguments and conflicts, inability to 'switch off', insomnia caused by such emotional turmoil.
Remedy: **White Chestnut**

LONELINESS

Reserved – may appear proud, aloof and unapproachable, enjoys own company, puts up an emotional barrier, bears grief in silence.
Remedy: **Water Violet**

Wrapped up in oneself – self-centred and self-concerned,

enjoys talking about self and own ailments, causes own loneliness, is draining on other people who therefore avoid the person concerned.
Remedy: **Heather**

Impatient – irritable, restless and fidgety, always in a hurry, cannot wait, intolerant of those who are slow.
Remedy: **Impatiens**

OVERSENSITIVITY TO INFLUENCES AND IDEAS
Jealousy, envy and hatred – feeling suspicious, bad-tempered and angry at other people.
Remedy: **Holly**

Being weak-willed and subservient – being unable to say 'no', easily exploited, a 'doormat' (may apply to children who always feel put upon and do what they are told).
Remedy: **Centaury**

Mental torment behind a brave face – cracking jokes about one's problems to conceal them, suffering deep-seated anxiety which has not been addressed and perhaps ending up having a breakdown and resorting to alcohol to 'dampen' feelings.
Remedy: **Agrimony**

Needing protection against change and outside influences – during the different stages of life such as marriage, divorce, giving birth, puberty, menopause, adjusting to transition and new surroundings.
Remedy: **Walnut**

DESPONDENCY OR DESPAIR
Lack of confidence – fear of failure, feelings of inferiority, particularly before exams or public performance.
Remedy: **Larch**

Feelings of being unable to struggle on – such as that experienced by a normally strong, steady worker who always strives to improve things and won't take a day off until there is a breakdown in health.
Remedy: **Oak**

Self-hatred, self-disgust – sense of uncleanliness, shame about certain ailments.
Remedy: **Crab Apple**

After-effects of shock – fright following an accident, grief or serious news, as in people who look visually 'dead' with no shine in the eyes or colour in the skin.
Remedy: **Star of Bethlehem**

Resentment – blaming people outwardly, embittered, exhibiting the 'poor old me' syndrome
Remedy: **Willow**

Self-reproach and guilt – blaming oneself inwardly. Being over-apologetic, with low self esteem.
Remedy: **Pine**

Overwhelmed by responsibility – feeling inadequate, unable to cope.
Remedy: **Elm**

Extreme mental anguish – despairing, crying silently, feeling that there is no light at the end of the tunnel or one is trapped in a suffering, unbearable anguish, inability to cope.
Remedy: **Sweet Chestnut**

OVERCARE FOR THE WELFARE OF OTHERS
Overenthusiasm – having strong feelings about various matters, being always on the go, unable to relax, pushing oneself too hard.
Remedy: **Vervain**

Intolerance – being critical of others, lacking empathy, being easily annoyed by other people's habits.
Remedy: **Beech**

Selfish possessiveness – over-protective, clinging, always needing to 'mother' someone and be the centre of attention.
Remedy: **Chicory**

Being domineering, inflexible – dominating, self-assured, having fixed opinions, being overpowering.
Remedy: **Vine**

Self-repression, self-denial – rigid-thinking, someone after an ideal life, looking for protection and purity, always needing to set an example to others, doing things to extremes.
Remedy: **Rock Water**

It is advisable to limit the choice of remedies to about six as too many taken together can cloud the issue and reduce their efficacy.

the
importance of
touch

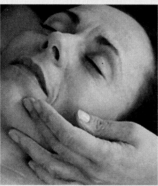

MASSAGE

- Aromatherapy
- Shiatsu
- Lymphatic drainage
- Ayurvedic medicine
- Reflexology
- Acupuncture

MASSAGE

We all need to be touched –
it shows us we are not alone.
The techniques described on
the following pages are some
of the ways we can touch
each other through massage
and related forms of healing.

As a foetus in the womb, our first impression was of touch
as it is the first of our senses to develop. It was a comfort to
us then and remains a comfort throughout our life. Our
sense of touch gives us our sense of reality. It is a mirror of
our emotions, making us tingle with excitement or feel
numb with shock or fear.

One of the most effective ways of touching another person in a
non-intrusive manner is through massage. Approximately 75
per cent of today's diseases are attributable to stress and
tension. Repressed emotions which often manifest themselves
in muscles and tendons can be released through massage,
thereby relaxing the whole mind and body.

During a massage a qualified therapist will usually devise a
programme to suit the individual. It could be a light relaxing
massage or, in cases of muscle tension, a deeper tissue
massage. It is not just the therapist who has to 'perform'; the
reaction of the client is equally important. For instance, during a
deep massage the client should not tense up through pain as
this will counteract any benefits. It is important to take low,
deep breaths which will generate relaxation, so improving the
quality of the treatment.

Massage should not be thought of as a luxury but as a way
of life. It does not have to be time-consuming either – a back,
neck and shoulder treatment needs only 15 to 30 minutes.

The spine is the core of the body's functions, with 33 pairs of
spinal nerves fanning out from the spinal cord. Each pair
stimulates the functioning of certain areas of the body and
massage increases this action.

Massage need not be expensive. Obviously clinics and beauty
salons vary in their charges, but cheaper treatments are available
at government-subsidized leisure centres. Why not sign up with
a friend to do a course in massage so that you will then be able
to treat each other, or use the techniques shown in this book.

BENEFITS

Massage can be beneficial in many of
the following ways. It can:
• Create deep relaxation and stimulate
circulation.
• Relieve muscle tension.
• Detoxify the body.
• Aid digestion.
• Increase the function of the
lymphatic system.

BEWARE

Massage should be avoided in cases of:
• Septic conditions.
• Varicose veins .
• Recent scar tissue.
• Cardiovascular conditions such as
angina, phlebitis and thrombosis.
• Pregnancy (avoid massage over the
abdomen unless by a therapist).
• Broken bones, bone cancer and
Hodgkin's disease.

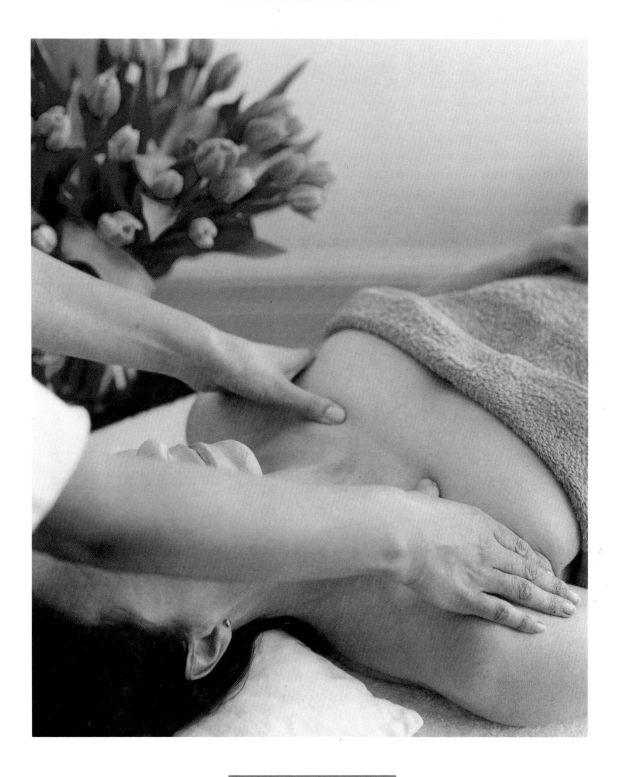

THE PRINCIPLE MASSAGE MOVEMENTS

EFFLEURAGE

It was Peter Henry Ling of Sweden (1776–1838) who founded the Swedish system of massage and introduced effleurage, pettrisage and many other techniques which are still taught today.

The term effleurage is derived from the French *effleurer*, meaning to skim over. It precedes all other massage movements as it is so relaxing, enabling the recipient to become acquainted with the therapist's hands.

Effleurage is performed mainly with the flat of the hand in long strokes. Pressure is emphasized on the upward stroke and the aim is to assist the nervous and lymph flow. Effleurage should follow the natural contour of the body, which is why it is important to use the whole hand.

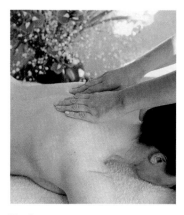

Back

❶ This stroke must be carried out on the muscle running up either side of the spine, not on the spine itself. Start with the hands together at the top of the back.

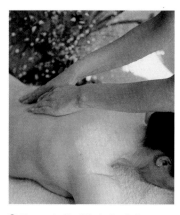

❷ Very gradually slide the hands down towards the lower back, leaning into the movement with your body weight.

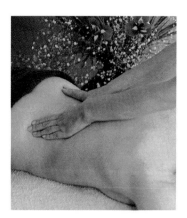

❸ When you have reached the lumbar area of the back, fan the hands out towards the sides of the waist. (This stroke is also beneficial for massaging the fronts and backs of the legs and the arms.)

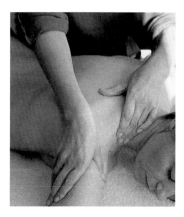

Shoulder

Make sure that the patient's arm is relaxed. Using the flat of one hand, follow the contour of the shoulder and the upper arm and move down towards the elbow and then up again.

THE PRINCIPLE MASSAGE MOVEMENTS

KNEADING

The word 'massage' may originate from the Greek for 'knead'. Kneading is one of the main massage movements and can be applied to many parts of the body, in particular to soft tissue areas.

Its action is similar to that of kneading bread, the object being to lift tissue away from the bone and roll it back, emphasizing pressure on the rolling action. The technique is very beneficial in breaking down fat, improving metabolism and eliminating waste products.

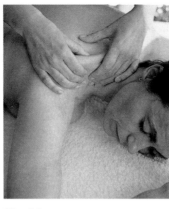

Shoulder

Pick up the shoulder muscles between fingers and thumb, squeezing and rolling. As this area often holds the most tension, do not be afraid to increase the pressure.

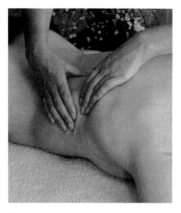

Waist

This movement is best worked on fleshy areas of the back, such as the sides, rather than the spinal area. It is also extremely effective on any fatty areas, such as buttocks and thighs.

PETTRISAGE

The term pettrisage originates from the French *petrir*, meaning to knead.

This movement is normally applied with the balls of the thumbs or fingers to soft tissue areas over bone. The squeezing action allows accumulated waste products to be eliminated. All these movements are good for tight calves and tight hamstrings.

It is advisable to keep the knee supported with a small cushion when working on the back of the leg.

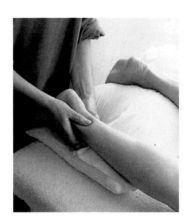

Calves

❶ Applying pressure with one thumb, start at the ankle and gradually slide the thumb up towards the calf muscle. If the calf muscle at any stage feels tight, hold the position, slightly circling the thumb.

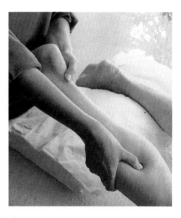

❷ Work up the centre of the calf and either side. Alternatively, petrissage can be carried out using both hands overlapping each other, with the top hand applying pressure on the lower one. (This movement is also effective on the back.)

THE PRINCIPLE MASSAGE MOVEMENTS

HACKING

Hacking is a very stimulating movement achieved using the edge of the hands. It generally improves circulation and the tone of muscular tissue. It is effective on buttocks, thighs and calves.

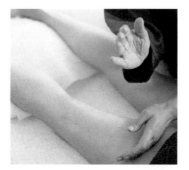

Backs of legs

❶ Keeping the wrists as relaxed as possible to avoid overtiring the neck and shoulders, hack against the backs of the legs in a fairly light and quick chopping movement.

WRINGING

The name 'wringing' perfectly describes itself: the movement literally 'wrings' tension from fleshy areas such as thighs and calves.

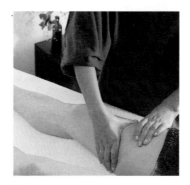

Thighs

❶ Hold the thigh between your thumbs and fingers, with one hand forward and the other back.

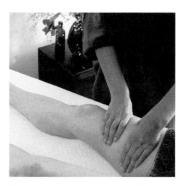

❷ Squeezing gently, pull one hand back and push forward with the other. Reverse the movement.

STOMACH

Of the techniques already mentioned, effleurage is perhaps the most effective movement for the sensitive stomach area. Applying pressure in long strokes with the whole hand, circle the waist in gentle movements. Stomach massage is particularly beneficial in relieving PMT and stomach aches.

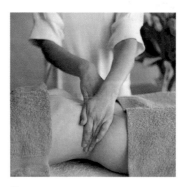

❶ Starting with both hands under the back, pull them up round the waist to the stomach, pressing gently.

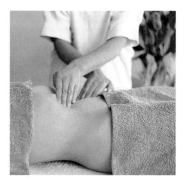

❷ Using alternate hands, describe large circles around the stomach, applying pressure with your fingers.

THE PRINCIPLE MASSAGE MOVEMENTS

FEET

Foot massage can also be greatly beneficial. Each foot contains around 7,000 nerve endings linked all over the body, and by massaging the feet it is possible to energize the whole body.

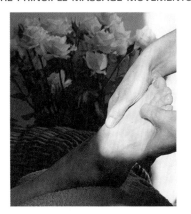

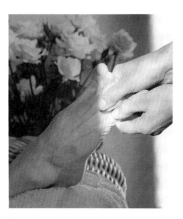

Tops of the feet

❶ Starting at the base of the foot, slide the thumb along the top of the foot to the toes, massaging between the tendons. Repeat on each tendon. This is beneficial for stimulating the lymphatic system and the chest area.

❷ Starting at the base of the toe, squeeze between fingers and thumb and pull up towards the tip. Repeat on each toe. This stimulating movement can help against headaches and sinus problems.

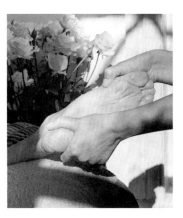

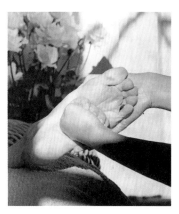

Arches of the feet

Cradle the heel in the left hand. Use the right thumb to slide from the base of the big toe down to the heel along the inside of the foot. This works on the spinal reflexes as well as stimulating the feet.

Soles of the feet

Using the knuckles, start from the ball of the foot and apply pressure in a sliding movement down to the base of the foot. This energizes the soles of the feet.

TECHNIQUE

Most facial massage movements are upwards towards the top of the head and outwards towards the side of the face: they should never drag the skin downwards. Care should be taken around the eyes, where the skin is particularly delicate.

FACIAL MASSAGE

There are around 12 major facial muscles and numerous underlying minor ones which are constantly used through expression. As we age these muscles, like those of the body, begin to lose their tone and start to sag. Facial muscles are often the first to show signs of the force of gravity, and it is this, rather than facial lines or wrinkles, which usually gives the appearance of ageing .

There are two ways to prevent or slow down this process: exercise of the facial muscles (see chapter four) and facial massage. Apart from stimulating the nerve endings and nourishing the skin by increasing the flow of oxygen through the blood, facial massage can also relieve tension, headaches and anxiety.

Pressure points of the face

There are a number of pressure points on the face which can contribute to healthy-looking skin when stimulated. They can easily be worked on at home in front of a mirror using the pad of the first or second finger.

stomach (helps abdominal cramps and indigestion)

headache relief

headache relief

sinuses

sinuses

eye-stress

eye-stress

kidney/adrenal

kidney/adrenal

sinuses

sinuses (nasal obstructions and allergies)

liver/lymphatic system

liver/lymphatic system

spleen/pancreas

pineal/pituitary

colon

colon

THE PRINCIPLE MASSAGE MOVEMENTS

HEAD AND SCALP MASSAGE

Head and scalp massage is a wonderful way of energizing the mind and the body and offers the bonus of promoting healthy hair growth.

Like the soles of the feet, the head has a number of reflex and acupuncture points. If pressure is applied correctly to them, it can benefit the whole body. It is always surprising how much tension is released after a treatment. Gently pulling the hair low down near the roots can also energize a sluggish system.

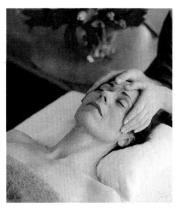

Forehead

❶ Place both thumbs parallel in the centre of the forehead, just above the eyebrows, with the fingers softly cradling the head.

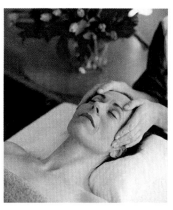

❷ Slowly slide the thumbs outwards, keeping the thumbs parallel. Follow the hairline around and down to the temples. Finally, change from thumbs to the middle fingers and gently circle the temples. Apply pressure as far as is comfortable.

CHEEK MASSAGE

These movements are easy to perform on oneself in front of a mirror – for instance, when applying facial moisturizer. They are particularly effective in relieving tension from sinus problems.

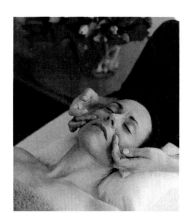

Cheekbones

❶ Using the edge of the middle finger, follow the contour of the cheekbones. Start on either side of the nose and gradually work around towards the ear, applying pressure quite firmly.

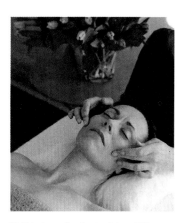

❷ This time using the tip of the middle finger, circle the whole cheekbone from the inside edge to the outside. Press quite firmly.

THE PRINCIPLE MASSAGE MOVEMENTS

JAW AND NECK MASSAGE

A youthful, healthy complexion does not emerge from a jar of cream; it lies in the condition of the muscle tissue. Massage, is one way, with diet and exercise, to boost the complexion and refine the areas prone to signs of ageing; the jaw and neck. It also relaxes tension in the jaw. For these exercises, it is easier to use a small amount of oil.

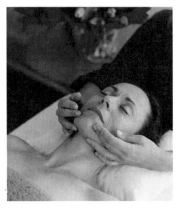

Jawline

Hold the chin between the third and fourth fingers and work out from the centre towards the ears. Press firmly, taking care not to press the throat.

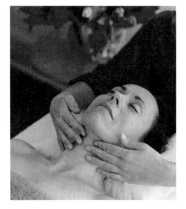

Neck

Using all the fingers, work from the throat out towards the ears, stroking very lightly and soothing the neck.

EAR MASSAGE

The Chinese are firm believers in auricular therapy and use around 100 acupuncture points in their treatments. However, a simple massage of the ears will stimulate the face and head area. Holding the earlobe between the thumb and index finger, make very small circular movements with the pad of the thumb. Work your way gradually up and around the fleshy part of the ear. The ears will redden – a mark of improved circulation, not pain!

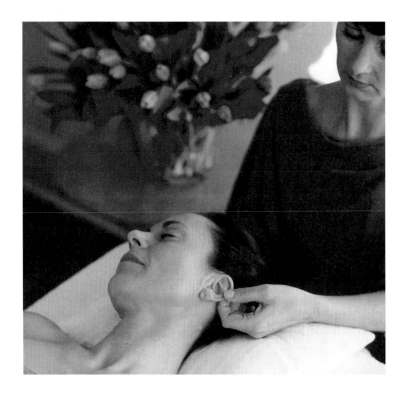

MASSAGE FOR BABIES AND CHILDREN

Massage is a natural way of increasing maternal bonding. In babies it can be very beneficial in reducing colic, constipation and colds, and it can also comfort and relax a baby who has difficulty sleeping.

Make sure you are in a warm environment. Using a light oil such as grapeseed or sweet almond for a massage, perform slow movements and exert gentle pressure. Avoid the face. In general do not use essential oils (see page 125), with the exception of a low dilution (1 drop in 10ml/1fl oz of carrier oil) of camomile, which is beneficial for colic. Mandarin can be used for constipation and lavender helps to soothe.

The techniques already described in this chapter can be used on babies and children. Massage should be enjoyable for them, but if they become restless and agitated it is best to stop.

MASSAGE FOR THE ELDERLY

Our need for touch does not diminish with age; in fact, for elderly people whose other senses are failing, leaving them feeling isolated and vulnerable, touch is a wonderful way to communicate love and affection. Just the simple act of holding someone's hand when they are feeling low can be healing.

Elderly people are often considered too fragile to massage, but even if their bodies are senescent they still need comfort and companionship. Massage is ideal for the elderly, especially if it is teamed with a certain amount of exercise, where possible, and a healthy diet. Even a gentle treatment can help circulatory problems (a simple massage can be a perfect way of warming cold hands and feet), arthritis and muscular stiffness, aiding relaxation and relieving high blood pressure.

In cases of immobility, massage can be carried out in a chair and applied through loose clothing. It is easy to massage the head, neck, shoulders and back if the recipient sits on a stool, astride a chair, or with the chair back to one side. If the recipient is mobile enough to lie on a massage table it is easy to treat any area of the body, clothed or unclothed. A little extra oil may be needed as dryness is often a problem with older skins.

BEWARE

• It is not advisable to work directly on arthritic joints if they are inflamed. However, where there is no inflammation, massage can certainly ease pain and stiffness.

• In cases of cardiovascular problems it is wise to consult a doctor before having or giving a massage.

Aromatherapy

BENEFITS

**Aromatherapy has proven beneficial
for relieving:**

• Stress.

• Anxiety.

• Depression.

• PMT.

• Menopausal problems.

• Insomnia.

• Allergies.

• Digestive problems.

• Muscular aches and pains.

The use of pure oils extracted from plants, flowers, trees and fruits adds a whole new dimension to massage. It is a truly 'holistic' therapy as, aside from their physical effects on the body, these essences have subtle influences on the mind and emotions which conventional medicines cannot always reach. During the past century synthetic chemicals have largely superseded essential oils in perfume and pharmaceuticals. However, the recent revival of aromatherapy has shown final recognition of the power of these oils. Today it is regarded as one of the most natural therapies.

Aromatherapy dates back thousands of years, when the oils were used in Egypt, China and Greece cosmetically and therapeutically and certain oils were used to embalm the dead. It was Avicenna, the great Arab physician, who discovered the aromatic purposes of the rose. By the thirteenth century lavender grew in England and in the early twentieth century its benefits were discovered accidentally by the French chemist René Maurice Gattefosse after he burned his hand while working in his laboratory. He plunged his hand into a bowl of lavender oil which he had thought was water and was amazed how quickly the pain disappeared and how fast the scar healed. He then decided to carry out research into other essential oils, which eventually led to the introduction of *aromatherapie* in France.

Essential oils are produced by tiny glands in the petals, stems, bark and wood of plants and trees, and also from the skin of many fruits. The oils are extracted through a process of distillation, expression (squeezing) or solvent extraction.

METHODS OF ABSORBTION

There are three ways in which essential oils may be absorbed by the body. Through:

Smell The sense of smell is the most immediate of our senses. When we smell an essential oil, the aromatic vapour dissolves into the moisture in the nose, stimulating the olfactory nerves. The fibres of these nerves are in direct contact with the limbic system of the brain, which is the basis of our feelings and emotions.

People are often unaware of the power of smell. Certain aromas can stimulate memories, recreate experiences, warn us of danger, arouse or comfort us. They can even induce hunger, which is why we often lose our appetite when we have a cold. Supermarkets with their own bakery that allow the aroma to waft into the store have found that bread sales increase.

The skin Skin is not impermeable and oils are easily absorbed into it as skin is lipophillic (contains fat) and oil is attracted to fat. Once the oil has penetrated the skin it passes through the lymphatic ducts and blood capillaries. In this way the aromatic particles pass into general circulation around the body.

Inhalation Deep inhalation, such as steam inhalation (over a bowl of hot water or a facial sauna) is beneficial for clearing sinuses, headaches and respiratory conditions.

USES OF AROMATHERAPY & ESSENTIAL OILS

Massage As well as possessing healing properties, essential oils bring a touch of luxury to a massage. The dilution should be one drop of essential oil to every 2ml of base (or carrier) oil. A blend of two or three essential oils is the usual composition in 5 or 6 ml of base oil.

Inhalation Put six to ten drops of essential oil in a bowl of hot water and sit comfortably, close to the bowl and with a towel over the head. Inhale for about 10 minutes. Facial saunas can also be used for this method.

Compresses Compresses are very effective in cases of pain, inflammation and swelling: use hot compresses for pain and cold compresses for swelling and inflammation. Dip a piece of lint or thin towelling or a face flannel into a basin of hot or cold water to which four to six drops of essential oil have been added. Wring out the compress and apply to the painful area. If using a hot compress, apply a new one once it has cooled. Cold compresses are beneficial for headaches, sprains and

BASE OILS

Grapeseed Suitable for all skin types.

Sweet almond Relieves itching, soreness, dry skin and inflammation.

Apricot kernel Suitable for all skins, especially prematurely aged, dry, inflamed or sensitive types.

Wheatgerm Beneficial for ageing skin, eczema and psoriasis. It is also useful to include if making up a blend of massage oil to as its stabilizing properties help to prolong the life of the blend. If there is an allergy to wheat, however, it is best to avoid this oil.

Jojoba Good for inflamed skin, psoriasis, eczema and prematurely aged skin.

Evening primrose Suitable for eczema, psoriasis and inflamed conditions.

Avocado Suitable for dry skin.

tennis elbow, and the addition of ice to the water is particularly helpful in the reduction of swelling.

Essence burners and light bulb rings Essence burners and rings which fit on to light bulbs are now widely available and are a wonderful way of scenting a room. A couple of drops of essential oil added to water in an essence burner or applied neat in a light bulb ring can be very beneficial to health. For asthma and hayfever, camomile and melissa are recommended.

In the bath Once the bath is run, add around six drops of essential oil and mix with the water so as not to leave a film on the surface. If you have sensitive skin you should take care.

On tissues, handkerchiefs and pillows Just a few drops of essential oil placed on a tissue and inhaled every so often will stimulate the mind. A few drops of the appropriate oil on the pillow can induce a restful sleep (see 'Insomnia', page 131).

BASE OILS

As well as acting as a carrier oil to essential oils in massage, many base oils can be used on their own. A few of them are described opposite, and there are numerous other vegetable oils which are beneficial provided they are cold-pressed.

PURCHASE AND STORAGE OF OILS

When buying essential oils it is advisable to buy high-quality unadulterated brands. Unless they are labelled 'pure essential oil', they have probably been diluted. They may be labelled 'aromatherapy oil', but this does not guarantee purity. The price of oils varies depending on the quality and process of extraction. Lavender oil, for example, is one of the cheaper oils in comparison with rose. It takes kilos of rose petals to produce a small amount of pure essential oil, whereas the same weight of lavender would produce ten times the quantity.

The oils should be stored in a cool dark place in dark glass bottles. The caps should be tight to prevent oxidation. If buying ready blended massage or bath oils, it is advisable to store them in a refrigerator once opened as this will preserve the quality for longer.

AROMATHERAPY AND PREGNANCY

Aromatherapy can be extremely advantageous both during and after pregnancy as this is a time of so many physical and emotional changes. In the Middle East it is common practice for a new mother to be massaged regularly after birth by the local midwife. Among the physical changes which can occur during pregnancy are: fluid retention, especially in the breast, leg and ankle area; haemorrhoids; varicose veins and thread veins; backache; constipation due to extra pressure on the lower abdomen; poor lymphatic drainage; nausea; stretch marks; and disturbed sleep. Emotionally women can feel anxious during the pregnancy and depressed and overtired after the birth through lack of sleep and hormonal changes, especially at the start of lactation.

Caution should be taken with rosemary and lavender as both these oils are emmenagogue, which means that they could bring on a period, and are therefore best avoided until after the sixth month. Before then they can be beneficial for backache if used in a low dilution and rose in particular is helpful for the emotional needs of an expectant mother.

To prevent stretch marks, use either mandarin or tangerine in a base oil of wheatgerm and massage the oils over the abdominal and hip area. For oedema (swelling) in the legs and ankles, geranium in a base oil of sweet almond or grapeseed, mixed in a low dilution and massaged upwards over the legs and ankles, can reduce the swelling. Camomile used in a low dilution is soothing to the digestive system. Lemongrass can stimulate the nervous system and is beneficial in cases of varicose veins and haemorrhoids. Ginger is often recommended for morning sickness, and neroli and rose are useful for post-natal depression.

The addition of essential oils to the bath during pregnancy can be very relaxing to the mind and body – but avoid overhot water. Massage by a therapist who is qualified for pregnancy treatment can be wonderfully comforting and, together with the support and empathy of the therapist, can be of enormous value during this important time in a woman's life.

WARNING

The following oils should never be used during pregnancy:

- Basil.
- Birch.
- Arnica.
- Cedarwood.
- Clary sage.
- Cypress.
- Fennel.
- Juniper.
- Marjoram.
- Peppermint.
- Rosemary.
- Sage.
- Thyme.

GLOSSARY OF THE PROPERTIES OF ESSENTIAL OILS

Analgesic relieves pain.

Anaphrodisiac diminishes sexual desire.

Anti-allergic reduces allergic sensitivity.

Anti-convulsive relieves convulsions.

Anti-depressant reduces depression.

Anti-inflammatory reduces inflammation.

Anti-rheumatic relieves rheumatic pain.

Anti-septic inhibits growth of bacteria.

Anti-spasmodic relieves muscle spasm.

Anti-toxic counteracts poisoning.

Anti-viral inhibits the growth of viruses.

Aphrodisiac stimulates sexual desire.

Astringent lightens the skin tissue.

Bechic relieves coughing.

Carminative prevents/relieves flatulence.

Cephalic stimulates the mind.

Cholagogue stimulates the production of bile.

Cicatrisant promotes the formation of scar tissue.

Deodorant counteracts body odour.

Depurative purifies the blood.

Digestive aids the digestion of food.

Diuretic increases urine secretion.

Emmenagogue induces menstruation.

Expectorant aids the removal of catarrh from the lungs.

Fermifuge reduces fever.

Fungicidal inhibits fungal growth.

Galactagogue induces the onset of lactation.

Hepatic acts as a liver tonic.

Hypotensive lowers blood pressure.

Laxative promotes bowel evacuation.

Nervine stimulates the nervous system.

Parturient induces labour.

Rubefacient produces warmth and redness to the skin when applied.

Sedative calms the nervous system.

Splenetic strengthens the spleen.

Stimulant increases activity of the body in general.

Sudorific promotes sweating.

Tonic has an uplifting and invigorating effect.

Uterine has a tonic action on the womb.

Vasoconstrictor causes small blood vessels to contract.

Vasodilator causes small blood vessels to expand.

Vermifuge expels intestinal worms.

Vulnerary helps wounds to heal.

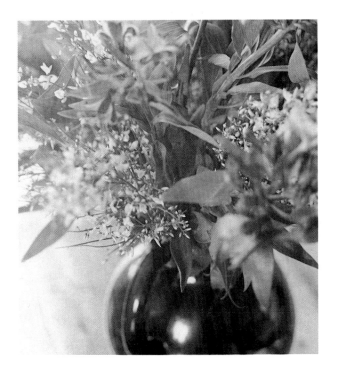

WARNING

Essential oils are very potent, making certain cautions vital:

- Do not take the oils internally.
- Do not apply directly to the skin, with the exception of lavender and tea tree oils in moderation.
- Keep the oils away from the eyes. Should an accident occur, wash with plenty of water.
- If taking homeopathic medicine, avoid using peppermint, black pepper, camphor and eucalyptus oils as they can counteract its efficacy. If in doubt, speak to your homeopathic doctor.

- If allergic to perfume, it is best to do a skin patch test first: blend one or two essential oils in a mild dilution (one drop of each essential oil in 10ml (1fl oz)of base oil), apply to the crease of the elbow and leave for 24 hours. If the skin does not react, you are not allergic to the oil(s).
- If sunbathing or using a sunbed, avoid using bergamot, lemon, orange and verbena oils as they can cause an allergic reaction to ultra-violet light.
- In cases of epilepsy, avoid sweet fennel, hyssop and wormwood oils.

- Hypertensives (sufferers from high blood pressure) should avoid rosehip, hyssop, sage and thyme oil.

Do not use any essential oils in cases of:

- Skin infections or septic area.
- Thrombosis and phlebitis, if using through massage.

In cases of cancer and treatment such as radiotherapy or chemotherapy, aromatherapy has proved a beneficial palliative. However it is best to check with a doctor first.

BENEFICIAL OILS FOR COMMON AILMENTS

AGEING SKIN
- **Frankincense** Rejuvenates
- **Geranium** Controls sebum
- **Sandalwood** For dry skin

ACNE
- **Lavender, Tea tree, Geranium** Anti-bacterial

ARTHRITIS
- **Camomile** Anti-inflammatory
- **Rosemary, Juniper** Detoxifying and beneficial in removing uric acid deposits
- **Black pepper, Eucalyptus, Marjoram** Warming

Massage any of these in a base oil directly on the affected area

CELLULITE
- **Geranium** Works on the hormonal system
- **Rosemary, Fennel** Diuretic and detoxifying

Massage any of these oils in a base oil directly on the affected area

CIRCULATION
- **Black pepper, Eucalyptus, Marjoram, Rosemary** Warming

CONSTIPATION
- **Basil, Fennel, Marjoram, Orange, Rosemary**
- **Camomile** For spasm in the colon as it has muscle-relaxant properties

COUGHS AND CATARRH
- **Eucalyptus and Camphor** For inhalation

CYSTITIS
- **Sandalwood, Cypress, Fennel, Juniper**

DE-HYDRATED SKIN
- **Camomile, Geranium, Rose, Sandalwood**

DEPRESSION
- **Rose, Geranium, Jasmine, Neroli, Lavender** For evening use
- **Bergamot, Basil, Grapefruit, Geranium, Clary sage, Rosemary**

ECZEMA
- **Camomile, Melissa**

FEET
- **Peppermint** Refreshes
- **Lemon grass** For dry skin

Use either in a foot bath or for massage

FLATULENCE
- **Basil, Fennel, Marjoram, Peppermint** For abdominal massage

HAEMORRHOIDS
- **Cypress, Juniper** Use in the bath. If constipation is the cause, use any of the oils listed under 'Constipation' for abdominal massage

HAIR
- **Rosemary** Dilute in sweet almond oil and use to massage the scalp to stimulate hair follicles and control sebum levels. For a final hair rinse add a few drops of rosemary for dark hair and camomile for fair hair

HEADACHES AND MIGRAINE
- **Lavender, Peppermint** Dab neat on each temple
- **Marjoram** Acts as a vasodilator (helps blood vessels to expand) if used in a cold compress on the forehead or in a warm compress on the back of the neck

IMMUNE SYSTEM
- **Geranium** Stimulates the adrenal cortex which plays a large part in the immune system as stress impairs resistance to infection
- **Black pepper, Lavender** Stimulate the spleen
- **Tea tree** One of the most powerful immune stimulants

INDIGESTION
- **Camomile, Fennel, Peppermint** Use either as an abdominal massage or drink in tea form

INFLAMMATION
- Camomile, Juniper, Rosemary

INFLUENZA
- Tea tree Use to support immune system
- Eucalyptus For sinus congestion
- Peppermint For headaches due to congestion

INSOMNIA
- Bergamot, Clary sage Use if the cause is mental worry
- Marjoram Very sedative
- Rose, Ylang ylang
Use all these oils in the bath at night or place a few drops on the pillow

LIBIDO
- Clary Sage, Jasmine, Neroli, Patchouli, Sandalwood, Rose, Ylang ylang Aphrodisiac
- Geranium Use if the cause is hormonal

LYMPHATIC SYSTEM
- Geranium, Juniper, Rosemary Use for massage

MENOPAUSE
- Camomile, Geranium, Rose For balancing the hormones to help loss of the feeling of femininity
- Clary Sage, Lavender, Neroli For balancing the emotions

- Fennel For its natural oestrogen content
All these oils should be used in a base of evening primrose oil for massage, otherwise add a few drops to the bath

MENSTRUAL PROBLEMS
- Camomile, Lavender For pain and cramps
- Clary Sage, Rose These are emmenagogue (induce menstruation) and therefore beneficial for infrequent periods
- Geranium, Rose Can regulate periods and are beneficial for heavy flow

OEDEMA (FLUID RETENTION)
- Cypress, Fennel, Juniper, Rosemary Diuretic and detoxifying
- Geranium Particularly good for swollen ankles and legs if used in massage

OESTROGEN
- Fennel A natural phyto-oestrol (plant hormone)
- Geranium, Rose Can stimulate the ovaries and adrenal glands, both of which are responsible for oestrogen production

OVERWEIGHT
- Cypress, Geranium, Lavender Rose, Ylang ylang Use if due to a hormonal imbalance

- Sandalwood Use if there is fluid retention
- Basil, Lavender, Orange, Rosemary Use if the nervous system needs stimulating (after illness, trauma or shock), for morning use
- Camomile, Lavender, Marjoram, Neroli, Ylang Ylang Use if the nervous system needs stimulating, for evening use

PMT
- Camomile, Geranium, Rose For depression and mood swings; use diluted in evening primrose oil

SORE THROAT
- Tea tree Gargle with two to four drops in a glass of water

STRESS
- Geranium Stimulates the adrenals, which become exhausted with severe stress
- Bergamot, Rosemary Uplifting
- Clary Sage, Jasmine, Neroli, Rose Relaxing

VARICOSE VEINS
- Black pepper, Juniper, Lavender, Rosemary Use in the bath
Caution: massage should not be applied directly on the veins but may be beneficial around the area affected

Shiatsu

BENEFITS

Shiatsu can help:

- Regulate hormonal functions.
- Strengthen the skin.
- Promote flexibility in the muscular tissues.
- Improve circulation of the bodily fluids.
- Stimulate the nervous system and the functioning of the internal organs.
- Alleviate back pain.
- Reduce migraines and headaches.
- Alleviate digestive problems.
- Assist cases of depression and insomnia.
- Normalize the menstrual cycle.
- Increase energy and relieve stress and stress-related symptoms.

For further information contact the Shiatsu Society which holds a register of practitioners (see page 219).

Originating as a folk medicine in Japan, shiatsu literally means finger *(shi)* pressure *(atsu)*. About 1,000 years ago Japan saw the arrival of Chinese medicine and this, combined with certain Chinese massage techniques used on various acupuncture points, formed the basis of shiatsu. It is now accepted as a medical treatment in Japan and its practitioners undergo extensive training in tsubo (point) therapy and diagnostic skills.

Shiatsu is always expanding, and new developments account for the various different styles of treatment available in the west, all of them based on the ancient theories.

How does shiatsu work?

If we were all 100 per cent healthy, our energy flow would be completely balanced. When we suffer illness, accident, or mental or physical trauma, our body's energy, or *ki* as it is known in Japan, becomes disturbed. Shiatsu aims to rebalance the quality and quantity of electro-magnetic energy which is distributed along the body's meridians (energy pathways) by stimulating certain tsubos (pressure points). When the *ki* is revitalized and flowing normally, it has a wonderful effect on all the body's systems, regenerating their functions and self-healing abilities.

The treatment entails working along the tsubos with the hands, knees or elbows, often including stretches to open up the meridians. Low-energy areas of the body are replenished by *ki* from high-energy areas, combining energy balancing with healing. A session will start with a consultation. Treatment, which usually lasts 50 minutes to an hour, is carried out on a special mat on the floor or the client can be seated. Loose clothing is advised as the client remains fully clothed. As with all holistic treatments there may be temporary 'healing reactions' such as headaches, sinus problems, or aching muscles. These are good signs of the body detoxifying, and drinking plenty of water will assist this cleansing process.

SHIATSU POINTS ON THE BODY

(FRONT) (BACK)

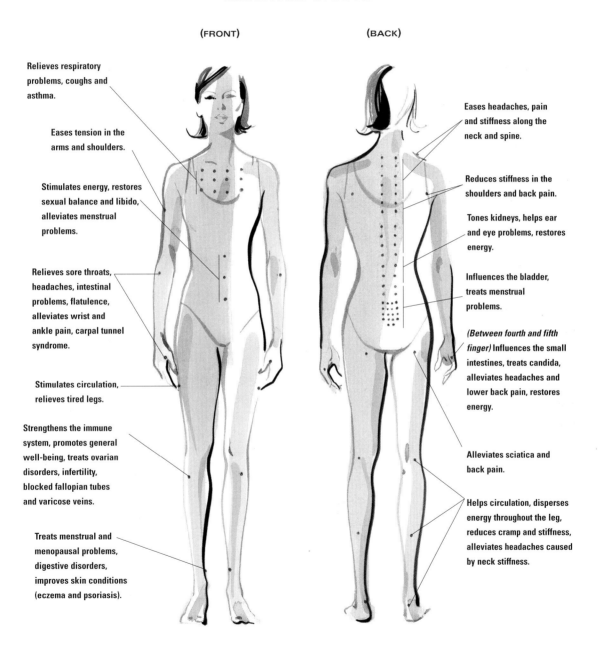

Relieves respiratory problems, coughs and asthma.

Eases tension in the arms and shoulders.

Stimulates energy, restores sexual balance and libido, alleviates menstrual problems.

Relieves sore throats, headaches, intestinal problems, flatulence, alleviates wrist and ankle pain, carpal tunnel syndrome.

Stimulates circulation, relieves tired legs.

Strengthens the immune system, promotes general well-being, treats ovarian disorders, infertility, blocked fallopian tubes and varicose veins.

Treats menstrual and menopausal problems, digestive disorders, improves skin conditions (eczema and psoriasis).

Eases headaches, pain and stiffness along the neck and spine.

Reduces stiffness in the shoulders and back pain.

Tones kidneys, helps ear and eye problems, restores energy.

Influences the bladder, treats menstrual problems.

(Between fourth and fifth finger) Influences the small intestines, treats candida, alleviates headaches and lower back pain, restores energy.

Alleviates sciatica and back pain.

Helps circulation, disperses energy throughout the leg, reduces cramp and stiffness, alleviates headaches caused by neck stiffness.

SHIATSU

Shiatsu uses touch to revitalize the body's energy, or *ki*, by stimulating various pressure points. These are known as tsubos. Common ailments such as colds, headaches and stress can be greatly alleviated by performing shiatsu on the tsubos. Here are ten principal points for you to massage yourself. Using the tips of your thumb or fingers, press gently as you breathe out. Repeat each exercise up to ten times.

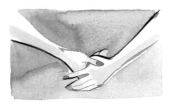

Toothaches, sore throats, headaches, flatulence, colds, sinus problems and pain in the upper body
This point lies between the thumb and forefinger on the back of the hand. Pressing the web of loose skin helps regulate the energy in the upper body.

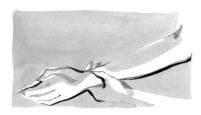

Colds and flu, stiff necks, congestion, coughs and headaches
This point lies on the inside of the arm just above where the wrist creases, on the same side as the thumb. Shiatsu on this point helps boost the lungs.

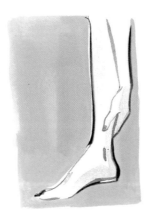

Period pains and problems, menopausal problems, pelvic problems, ankle pain, insomnia and digestive disorders
This point lies four finger-widths above the ankle bone, on the inside of the leg just behind the tibia.

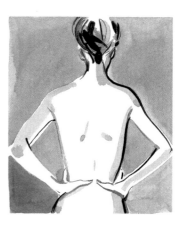

Lower back pain, sluggish kidneys, ear and eye problems
This point lies either side of the spine between the second and third lumbar vertebra. To locate it, wrap your hands around your waist with your thumbs two finger-widths apart on the spine.

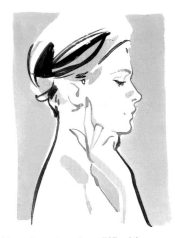

Earaches, hearing difficulties and tinnitus
This point lies just in front of the ear between the middle of the ear and the jaw.

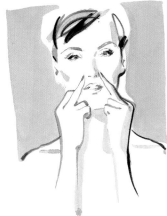
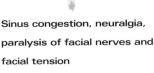

Sinus congestion, neuralgia, paralysis of facial nerves and facial tension
This point lies on either side of the base of the nose.

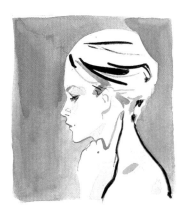

Headaches, colds, tension, eye disorders, dizziness and vertigo
This point lies just below the base of the skull in the hairline, in the hollow between the back and side neck muscles.

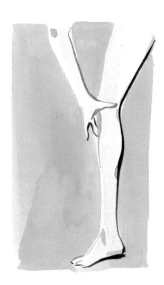

Muscle cramp and stiffness, circulation in the leg
This point lies in the centre of the crease on the back of the knee.

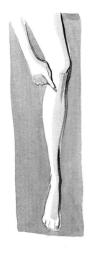

Indigestion, loss of appetite, nausea, tiredness, poor immune system, aching legs
This point lies four finger-widths below the knee. To locate it, feel for the depression beside the tibia bone.

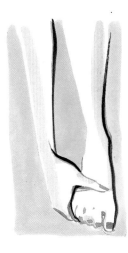

Stress, headaches, dizziness and muscle cramps
This point lies on the top of the foot where the bones of the first and second toes meet.

Lymphatic drainage

Manual lymphatic drainage (MLD) is a lighter form of massage which stimulates one of the body's most vital waste disposal units, the lymphatic system, by increasing the flow of lymph throughout the body. Lymph is a colourless fluid found outside the cells. In a normally functioning lymphatic system this fluid travels around the body, acting as a drainage system for the circulation, and is also the seat of our immune system.

Unlike the vascular system, the lymph system has no pump to assist the lymph in its journey around the body, so it relies upon muscle contraction. In an active person who exercises regularly this works perfectly well, but anyone with a sedentary lifestyle will probably be prone to a sluggish lymph system. For this reason it is important to keep the system stimulated, especially as we grow older.

The signs of a sluggish system are: tiredness, skin disorders, cellulite, bags under the eyes, low resistance to illness, swollen joints and rheumatic conditions, tension in the muscles and circulatory problems.

MLD uses delicate pumping movements which encourage the flow of lymph towards the lymph nodes, the little reservoirs situated around the body which act as filters to prevent infection spreading into the bloodstream. Although the treatment feels light, it is effective.

MLD is particularly beneficial after pregnancy. In France it is practised so frequently that it is now available on their national health service. Together with skin brushing, attention to the correct exercise and diet, MLD can help a number of degenerative conditions. Many people are also using MLD as a beauty treatment as it has the ability to tighten the skin, reduce puffiness, stretchmarks and cellulite. By reducing toxins from the body, it also has a general regenerative effect on the skin.

It is important to ensure your therapist is fully qualified in MLD as it is a specialized training which differs from other massage techniques. (See page 219 for useful addresses.)

Ayurvedic medicine

Ayurveda, which in Sanskrit means knowledge (*ayur*) of life (*veda*), is a traditional medicine from India. Over the past 4,000 years it has been developed through religious soul-searching and meditation by the *rishis*, holy wisemen. It shares similar theories to traditional Chinese medicine relating to energy points, pulse diagnosis and herbal remedies.

One of the ayurvedic philosophies is that everyone and everything in the universe is made up of three basic elements called doshas. These doshas are compared to the workings of the wind, sun and moon respectively and in Sanskrit are called vata, pitta and kapha. It is the mixture of doshas which creates an individual's make-up.

VATA is likened to the wind and controls the central nervous system. Vata people are often nervous and constantly on the go. Too little sleep, emotional outbursts, irregular meals and general overexertion can all cause vata imbalance.

PITTA is linked to the sun or force of heat, a source of energy which controls the digestive system and all biochemical processes. Indigestion, constipation, acidity and emotional fearfulness can cause a pitta imbalance.

KAPHA is the bioforce for growth and structure of the body, and the balance of tissue fluid. The common cold is signified by too much kapha, and mucus-associated problems are usually caused by a kapha imbalance. People who do not exercise and tend to fall asleep during the day are kapha types.

Ayurvedic practitioners begin by finding out about the diet, lifestyle and medical history of the client. They may take your pulse, examine your tongue, eyes, skin and possibly your urine and saliva to determine your individual constitution, or *prakruti*. Once your type is established, it is easier to work on your exercise, nutritional and psychological needs. They will suggest remedies from herbs, vegetables or minerals, dietary regimes or practical help such as massage, breathing exercises, yoga, meditation, steam baths, oil treatments and internal cleansing.

BENEFITS

Ayurveda focuses on removing the cause of illness rather than treating the symptoms, with the aim of strengthening the immune system and restoring energy. Used in conjunction with a healthy diet, exercise and meditation, it is easier to achieve harmony within the mind and body. It can benefit the following:

• Digestive problems.

• Asthma.

• Diabetes.

• Eczema and psoriasis.

• Arthritis.

• Ulcers.

• Stress and tension.

• Hormonal imbalance.

Many orthodox doctors are now practising ayurvedic medicine in Britain as well as numerous Indian trained practitioners. For further information contact the Association of Ayurvedic Practitioners (see page 219).

Reflexology

BENEFITS

There are a great number of conditions for which reflexology has proved beneficial:

- **Back pain.**
- **Sinus problems.**
- **Digestive conditions (constipation, IBS and so on).**
- **Weak immune system.**
- **Headache and migraine (including those caused by hormonal problems such as PMT, menopause and thyroid conditions).**
- **Stress and tension.**
- **Depression.**
- **Pregnancy.**

Originating in China and Egypt thousands of years ago, reflexology is a therapy which uses pressure on the feet or hands based on the principle that they contain reflex areas corresponding to different parts of the body. By stimulating these various reflexes it is possible to enhance the inherent healing abilities of the body. Reflexology is much more than a remedial treatment to be applied only during illness; in fact many people enjoy regular sessions to give the body an 'MOT'.

During a lifetime, the feet carry an individual the equivalent of five times around the earth. They are a very important, though often neglected, part of our anatomy and their structure has a definite bearing on our health. For example, tight shoes or heels which are too high can have a profound effect on posture and spinal alignment.

There are around 7000 nerve endings in each foot, each one connecting to a different area of the body (see below). Through

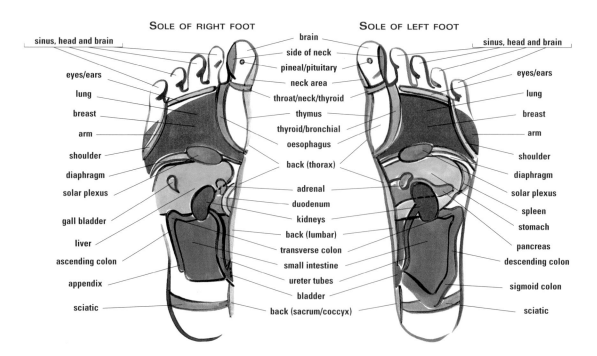

SOLE OF RIGHT FOOT	SOLE OF LEFT FOOT

sinus, head and brain

brain
side of neck
pineal/pituitary
neck area
throat/neck/thyroid
thymus
thyroid/bronchial
oesophagus
back (thorax)
adrenal
duodenum
kidneys
back (lumbar)
transverse colon
small intestine
ureter tubes
bladder
back (sacrum/coccyx)

eyes/ears
lung
breast
arm
shoulder
diaphragm
solar plexus
gall bladder
liver
ascending colon
appendix
sciatic

sinus, head and brain
eyes/ears
lung
breast
arm
shoulder
diaphragm
solar plexus
spleen
stomach
pancreas
descending colon
sigmoid colon
sciatic

reflexology, energy is increased along the meridians (the body's energy channels), unblocking areas of congestion which may be the cause of an imbalance in a particular organ or gland. To a reflexologist, a person's feet represent a mirror of the body.

Although it is more beneficial to be treated by a qualified practitioner, it is possible to practise on yourself at home using thumb or finger pressure on the relevant reflexes shown on the chart below.

COMMON AILMENTS AND THEIR REFLEXES

Condition	Reflex	Condition	Reflex
Anaemia	Spleen, liver	Haemorrhoids	Diaphragm, adrenals, rectum, sigmoid flexure, lower spine
Ankles (swollen)	Kidneys, adrenal, lymph system	Headaches	Whole spine, all glands, liver, all toes
Abdominal bloating	Stomach, diaphragm, intestines, liver	Menopause (hot flushes)	All glands, reproductive system, diaphragm, uterus
Asthma	Chest/lung, adrenals, diaphragm, ileocaecal valve	Migraine	Whole spine, diaphragm, big toes, pituitary, intestines
Breast lumps (benign)	Chest/lung, lymph system, pituitary	Morning sickness	All glands, diaphragm, stomach, ovaries, uterus
Backache	Spine	Ovarian cysts	Fallopian tubes
Cramps (foot and leg)	Hip/knee, hip sciatic, lower spine, adrenals, parathyroids	Motion sickness	Ear reflex, neck, diaphragm, spine
Cystitis	Kidneys, bladder, ureter, ureters, lower spine, adrenals	Sciatica	Hip, lower spine, sciatic area
		Sore throat	Adrenals, cervical region
Dry skin	Thyroids, adrenals	Stress	Diaphragm, all glands
General fatigue	Adrenals, diaphragm, all glands, whole spine	Thyroid	Pituitary, thyroid, adrenals

Acupuncture

BENEFITS

Acupuncture has a wide range of benefits, including conditions such as:

- Digestive problems.
- Neurological conditions, e.g. sciatica.
- Circulatory problems.
- Auto immune disorders such as rheumatoid arthritis, ME and multiple sclerosis.
- Gynaecological problems.
- Lung congestion.
- Allergies.
- Emotional problems.
- Skin conditions.
- Addictions – smoking, drugs, alcohol etc.
- Sleep disorders.

Literally translated from the Latin *acus* (needle) and *punctura* (puncture) acupuncture is part of the traditional system of Chinese medicine which uses needles to treat various diseases and ailments. It has been practised in China for around 3,500 years and is believed to have originated from the observation that soldiers who were wounded by arrows during battle sometimes mysteriously recovered from other long-standing health problems. The first medical textbook on acupuncture, *The Yellow Emperor's Classic of Internal Medicine* was produced in China around 4,000 BC. Its basic text is still as relevant today as it was thousands of years ago.

By the early twentieth century some British doctors began using acupuncture for the relief of pain and fever. By the Second World War western medicine was being used in China, and today both traditional Chinese and western medicine are often practised side by side.

Acupuncture is based on the principle that we all have energy or *Qi* (pronounced 'chi'), circulating around our bodies through invisible energy channels called meridians. Physical, emotional and environmental disorders can, however, alter the flow of energy, speeding it up, slowing it down, diverting it to the wrong area or even completely blocking it. Our way of living influences our *Qi*: if we eat a healthy balanced diet, exercise regularly and breathe in clean air, we enhance our store of energy; if we do not, we deplete it. Illness is a deficiency of the elemental energies in the body, creating an energy imbalance.

By inserting fine needles into certain points along the meridians, acupuncture can unblock, increase or decrease, the energy, so correcting the imbalances which are affecting our health. The important acupuncture points are located on the 14 meridians, each one named after the organ it represents, such as the heart, kidney, liver, gallbladder, lungs, stomach, spleen, small intestine and large intestine or colon. On modern acupuncture charts there are almost 2,000 points.

The Chinese also view the balance of *yin* and *yang* as an important part of harmony within the body. Universally there are five elements – wood, fire, earth, water and metal/air. Everything is controlled by the opposite forces of *yin* or *yang*. *Yin* is the female force representing darkness, coldness, dampness and swelling and is passive and tranquil, while *yang* is the male force representing light, heat, dryness and contraction.

Each of the body's meridians is described by an element and an energy. For example, the heart is said to be *yin* and fire. During a consultation the acupuncturist will determine, through observation and questioning, whether there is too much or too little of a particular element or energy in your body. The therapist usually feels the six subtle 'energy pulses' on each wrist in order to assess any disturbances in energy flow or malfunctioning of internal organs. He/she will usually look at the tongue and the condition of skin, eyes and hair. Once all the necessary information has been acquired, the acupuncturist is able to determine the specific imbalance(s) and the points that need treating.

When the needles are inserted, some people feel a slight prick. Once the needles are in, however, there is usually very little feeling. In most cases the needles will have been machine-sterilized; otherwise disposable ones are used. They may be left in for just a few minutes or as long as half an hour. Some practitioners use moxibustion as a way of heating the needle gently. There are two methods: the first involves filling a roll of paper about 15cm/6in long with moxa wool (prepared from the leaves of common mugwort), lighting it and holding it above the acupuncture point where the needle has been inserted. The second involves placing small cones of moxa on the heads of the needles and then lighting them. With this method the needle is sometimes inserted through a piece of cardboard to prevent any hot ash from falling on to the patient's skin.

You can sometimes get acupuncture on the National Health Service, and some doctors practise acupuncture themselves or their surgery may employ a practitioner. Alternatively they may be able to refer you to a qualified acupunturist.

WHERE TO GO

There are two main groups of acupuncturists:
• Medical acupuncturists. These are qualified doctors who have had extra training in acupuncture and use it alongside their orthodox treatments.
• Traditional acupuncturists. These are usually not qualified doctors but will have completed a course lasting from two to four years, which includes studying aspects of western medicine such as anatomy.
For details of professional organizations, see page 219.

exercise for longevity

EXERCISE
- How to exercise
- Pregnancy and exercise
- Arthritis and exercise
- Exercising after a stroke
- Methods of exercise
- Brain fitness
- Exercising the face

EXERCISE

Staying active and
keeping fit is a crucial part
of retaining our independence
and general feeling of
wellbeing as we get older.
In this chapter we will
explore the many ways
exercise can contribute to this.

Physical activity should be a natural part of life, not just something that we experience as children. In childhood we think nothing of running around expending seemingly endless energy in play or on the sports field. When we become adults, however, this physical activity declines because of sedentary jobs and too many home comforts. Only a few decades ago there were no washing machines, dishwashers, vacuum cleaners, hedge trimmers, grass trimmers, remote controls or mobile phones. There were many fewer cars on the road, and in general people walked more. Today the average British person spends 26 hours a week sitting in front of the television. We are becoming less fit as we grow older and by not exercising we are depriving ourselves of health and additional years of life.

BENEFITS

The numerous benefits of exercise include:

• Strengthening the vigilance of the immune system.
• Producing endorphins, the body's natural pain killers.
• Relieving depression.
• Increasing energy.
• Raising HDL levels in the blood, thereby balancing cholesterol.
• Reducing the risk of heart disease and stroke.
• Increasing blood circulation.
• Increasing metabolic rate.
• Controlling body weight.
• Increasing body co-ordination.
• Giving you a feeling of achievement and boosting confidence.

According to Hippocrates, 'All parts of the body which have a function, if used in moderation and exercised in labours in which each is accustomed, become thereby healthy, well developed and age more slowly. But if unused and left idle, they become liable to disease, defective in growth and age quickly.' This could be succinctly summed up today as: 'Use it or lose it'. If you compare the human body to, say, a car, consider how it would feel if it were left standing over a long period of time. Like a car it would deteriorate. As the body is a far more complex and wondrous construction than any car, this comparison emphasizes the importance of regular exercise, and if you have been inactive for a long time it is especially important that you begin to build up gradually.

An average person's lean body mass declines with age and the rate of decline accelerates after the age of 45. Muscles also become shorter with age and if inactive they can contract, causing stiffness, aches and pains. This can then lead to the onset of many problems such as headaches, rheumatism, backache and joint inflammation.

Exercise should be enjoyable; it should never be thought of as a chore, but as something that will give you zest and vitality. If it becomes boring, change your form of exercise. You may like to exercise in a group – perhaps joining a class or gym – so that it becomes a social activity where you can meet and become acquainted with other people. Get motivated rather than making one of the typical excuses – 'I can't fit into my leotard any more' or 'I ached all over when I tried it before' or 'I've got a bad knee/hip/back'. Once you've been to the gym or started exercising you will be able to fit into that leotard and, yes, you probably did ache after the first time because your muscles had forgotten what it felt like to be worked.

Remember that muscles and joints deteriorate through a period of inactivity, and provided the exercise is not detrimental to the afflicted area of your body, it will actually benefit it.

WHICH KIND OF EXERCISE?

When deciding on what kind of exercise would be most suitable for you, it is important to understand the three main types of exercise, namely aerobic, anaerobic and muscle strengthening.

AEROBICS

Aerobic is the term used to define the function of cells that need oxygen to 'burn' food in order to create energy. Aerobic exercises get the heart pumping faster. When you exercise, your muscles need extra oxygen and nourishment. Energy comes from the breakdown of sugars in the muscle tissue, and its energy production depends on how much oxygen reaches the muscle cells through the bloodstream. Exercise will make the heart muscle more supple, enabling contractions to be more powerful and forcing out more blood.

Running, cycling, swimming, jogging, dancing, skipping, step classes and sport are all forms of aerobic exercise, but it is important to stress here that you should get slightly out of breath for these types of exercise to be fully aerobic. Slow strolling or slow swimming are not aerobic, while running is. Your pulse rate should rise with aerobic exercise.

CAUTION

Consult your medical doctor for advice on the safest methods of exercising if you suffer from any of the following conditions:
- High blood pressure.
- Heart disease.
- Chest pain.
- Back pain.
- Diabetes.
- Arthritis.

BENEFITS

Aerobic exercise is particularly effective for:
- Increasing oxygen supply to the muscles.
- Increasing stamina.
- Increasing metabolic rate.
- Controlling body weight.
- Increasing body temperature.
- Increasing lung power – weak lungs encourage chest infections as there is more of a chance of bacteria build-up.

Twenty minutes to half an hour, two or three times a week, is a good average time for aerobic exercise depending on your level of fitness and health in general. Bowls and golf can improve flexibility in arms and shoulders but can put a strain on a bad back.

ANAEROBICS

Anaerobic exercise takes place during the first phase of any physical exercise, or during any exercise which is performed for a short time, such as weight-lifting or sprinting.

In general any continuous exercise which exceeds 20 minutes in length becomes aerobic. Weight training performed in short bursts is anaerobic, whereas if it is performed in a manner such as circuit training it can become more aerobic than anaerobic.

MUSCLE STRENGTHENING THROUGH WEIGHT-TRAINING

There are numerous ways of muscle strengthening, and the use of weights actually works the heart to a certain degree so it also falls into the aerobic category. Working with resistance machines at a gym or using hand or ankle weights at home, you are able to isolate muscle groups. Shoulders, arms, calves, thighs, buttocks and hips, stomach and abdominals can all be strengthened according to your own desire.

If you haven't exercised before or are particularly unfit, it is best to start with a supervised programme as lifting weights which are too heavy too suddenly could raise your blood pressure. It is also extremely important that you do not arch your back through straining to lift weights.

It has been proved that no area of the population can benefit more from exercise, and muscle strengthening exercise in particular, than senior citizens. One eight-week study in America of 87–96-year-old women confined to a nursing home showed that resistance exercise tripled their muscle strength and increased the muscle size by ten percent. Much of the loss of muscle that occurs as we age must therefore be not only preventable but also reversible.

BENEFITS

Anaerobic exercise helps:

• Increase lymphatic circulation.

• Speed up gastro-intestinal functioning.

• Reduce diabetes, as the cells become more receptive to insulin.

• Prevent disability.

BENEFITS

Muscle strengthening exercises can be used to:

• Increase muscle strength.

• Increase bone density, an important factor around the time of the menopause in the prevention of osteoporosis.

• Build tendon and ligament strength.

• Build muscle tissue, and so provide a greater capacity for the storage of glycogen, which is needed for energy.

• Build new muscle fibres, thus regenerating lost muscle power.

How to exercise

Once you have made the decision to exercise, the most important thing is not only that you enjoy it, but that you learn to do it in the most effective way.

When you start off, there is no need to exercise for more than about 20 minutes, and only when you are comfortable with this, can you gradually build up to longer sessions, otherwise you will end up sore and stiff. Obviously if you are very fit, longer and more frequent sessions are fine, but you should aim to build up to 20 or 30 minutes' fairly strenuous exercise two or three times a week. The key is to maintain a regular programme. If, as many people do, you find it difficult to put aside time for exercise, there are many subtle ways you can incorporate it into the average working day. Why not use the stairs instead of the lift, or walk part of the way to work. During the day try not to sit for longer than an hour without getting up to stretch the body, and encourage yourself to be more active generally.

Many people find that the easiest way to follow an exercise routine, at least in the beginning, is at home, so the exercises on the following pages have been designed with this in mind. You can perform them virtually anywhere, on your own or with a friend for moral support, all you need is a mat or thick towel. Most of the exercises are low impact aerobic and stretching exercises, which should lengthen the muscles without jerking them. Before stretching, the muscle fibres lie dispersed in a rather disorganized way throughout body tissues, but when they are stretched for a while, they line up with one another, which allows easier separation and a lengthening of the tissue.

If you suffer from back problems, it is advisable to do stretching exercises lying on your back, making sure that it is well supported to take the weight off the spine. When stretching it is also a good idea to loosen the joints, such as those in the shoulders, knees, hips, ankles and neck first to increase their blood supply, and make the stretching easier.

TAKE CARE

To get the most out of your exercise:

• Always warm up and cool down sufficiently.

• Invest in a good pair of supportive trainers, especially if you are running outside.

• If you have eaten a heavy meal, wait at least one and a half hours before exercising.

• Never exercise to the point of exhaustion.

• Choose a regular prgramme and stick to it.

• Don't exercise if you have a fever.

WARM-UP EXERCISES

Before any form of exercise, it is essential that you warm up the body. Just five to ten minutes of warming-up exercises can reduce the risk of injuries.

As you progress to the more intensive stretching exercises try to feel the muscles lengthen but not jar. While breathing normally, hold each stretch for 30 to 60 seconds, stretch a tiny bit further, and for longer and then relax. Most exercises should be repeated five to ten times increasing to a maximum of 20.

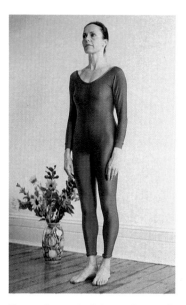

For a good stance in all the exercises stand straight up, keeping shoulders in line with hips, feet slightly apart and eyes ahead.

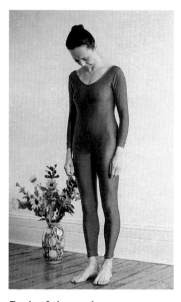

Back of the neck
Slowly lower the chin towards the chest. Keep the shoulders relaxed.

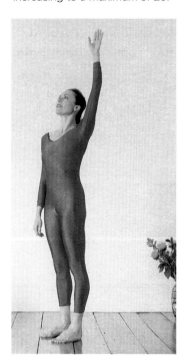

Side of body
Reach up as high as you can with the left arm and look up. Repeat to the right.

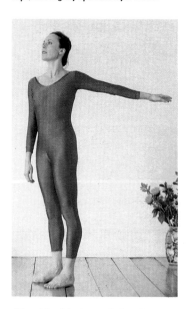

Shoulder blade and chest
Reach back at shoulder height with the left arm. Repeat to the right.

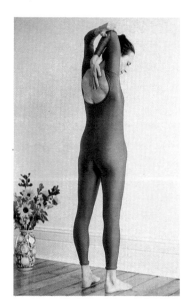

Triceps and shoulder (loosens)
Bend the right arm behind the head, and pull the elbow down gently. Repeat to the left.

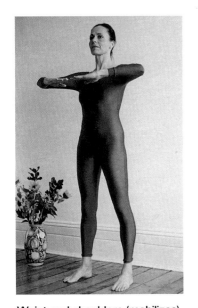

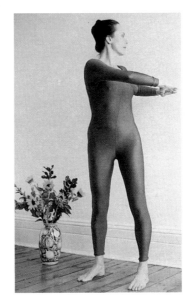

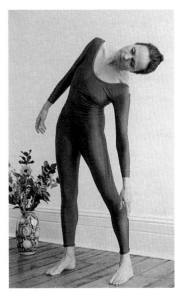

Waist and shoulders (mobilizes)

❶ Stand with feet and hips in line, arms raised so fingers are in line with middle of the chest.

❷ Keeping the arms at shoulder level, twist from the waist round to the left without moving your hips. Repeat to the right.

Side of waist

Bend to the left keeping the hips still. The hand leads down the leg. Repeat to the right.

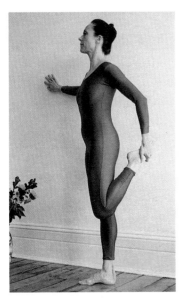

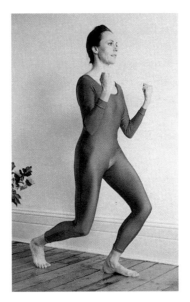

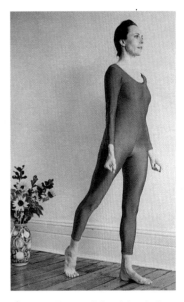

Front of thigh

Standing on right leg, hold left ankle in left hand and pull back. Repeat with right leg.

Front of thigh, shin (opposite legs)

❶ With right leg directly behind hip, bend both knees and bring the arms up in front of the body.

❷ Keeping legs parallel, straighten both knees so heel of back foot is still raised, and lower the arms. Repeat to both sides.

FLOOR EXERCISES

These exercises are great for the particular areas which women are anxious to keep in shape – the 'legs, bums and tums'. Each exercise should be done five to ten times, building up to more as you feel your muscles getting stronger. Always relax your back well into the floor and remember to inhale in the relaxed position and exhale during the exertion.

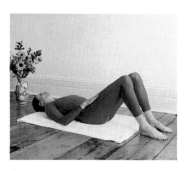

Stomach

❶ Lie flat on the floor with knees bent, feet in line with hips and back relaxed into the mat.

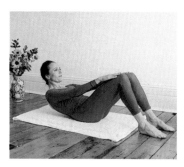

❷ Lift head and shoulders off the mat, and reach with arms towards the knees, pulling the stomach in to the spine. Hold then relax.

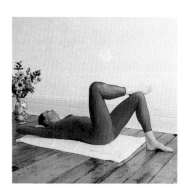

Stomach and waist

❶ Place the right ankle across the left knee, and gently support head with hands.

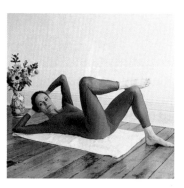

❷ Keeping the stomach flat, push the left elbow towards the right knee. Repeat to each side.

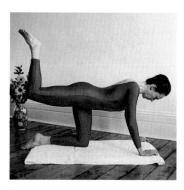

Buttocks and backs of thighs

❶ Arms in line with shoulders, kneel on the left leg, and raise the right leg to a 90° angle.

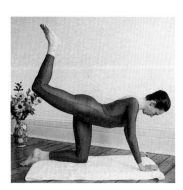

❷ With a flat stomach and keeping the head in line with the back, lift the right leg up from the hip a few inches. Repeat to each side.

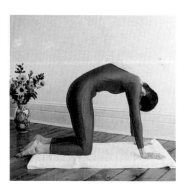

Spine (mobilises)

❶ Kneel on all fours and curve the spine, keep a flat stomach and pull the head under.

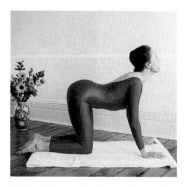

❷ From the same kneeling position, arch the back and roll the head slowly up. Arms should stay a shoulder width apart.

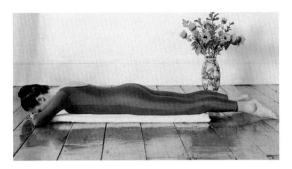

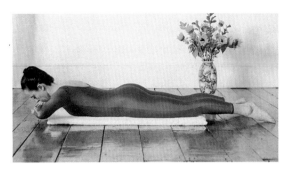

Back (strengthens)

❶ Lie face down on a mat, with hands under the forehead and palms facing downwards.

❷ Pulling the stomach in, and keeping the shoulders down into the back lift the upper chest and head off the mat. Do not pull on your neck.

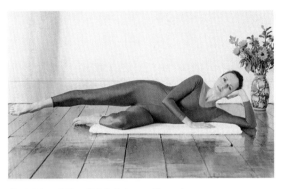

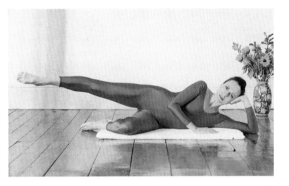

Outside of the thigh (strengthens)

❶ Lie on the left side, with the left leg bent in front of you, and the right leg extended in line with the hip a few inches above the floor.

❷ Using the left hand to support the head and the right for balance raise right leg four inches, keeping it straight and turned inwards from hip. Keeping a strong stomach, lower the leg. Repeat to each side.

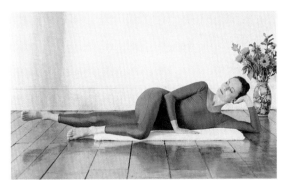

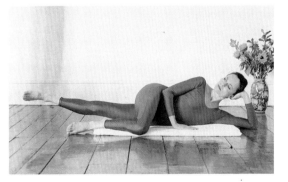

Inside of the thigh (strengthens)

❶ Now with a flexed foot extend the left leg just off the floor in line with the hip and bend the right leg over in front of the body.

❷ Raise the left leg up from the top of the inner thigh four inches and try to reach out from the heel as though lengthening your thigh. Keeping a strong stomach, lower the leg. Repeat to each side.

COOL DOWN EXERCISES

At the end of any exercise programme, you must always allow time for cooling down. Not only does this prevent excessive stiffness and jarring of the muscles, but it also allows the system to slow down gradually. This is especialy important after vigorous aerobic exercise. As well as performing the cool down exercises shown here, you may also find it beneficial to repeat some of the warm-up and stretching exercises from page 148 and 149. Remember to do everything as gradually as possible – there should be no rushed movements at all.

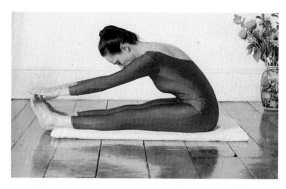

Hamstrings, neck and spine Sit on the mat with legs outstretched, reach towards flexed toes and keep the shoulders down.

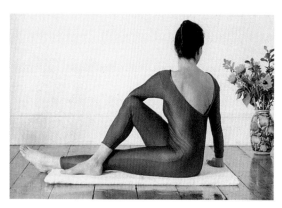

Waist Bend right leg across left, put left elbow on right knee and twist right from waist keeping hips square. Hold and relax. Repeat to other side.

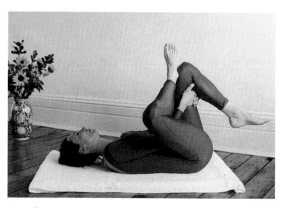

Buttock Lie on your back with the right ankle across the front of the left knee. Clasp hands behind the left thigh and pull it towards the chest.

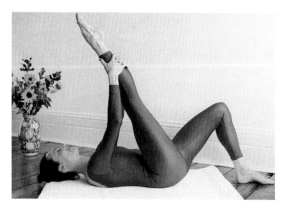

Hamstring ❶ Lie on your back with left leg bent. Clasp hands round lower right leg and pull it towards the chest keeping knee straight.

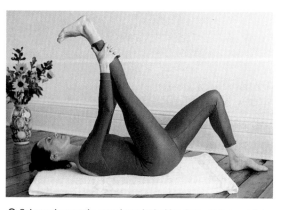

❷ Relax and repeat the exercise to both sides, first with toes pointed and then with foot flexed to intensify the stretch.

Pregnancy and exercise

Being pregnant, is not a reason to give up exercise. In fact, at this stage of life, it can be particularly benefical. Swimming can be particlarly beneficial for both mother and baby since it oxygenates the blood and this in turn nourishes the baby and creates a healthier environment.

EXERCISE DURING PREGNANCY

The birth in itself will be quite a strenuous exercise, requiring increased stamina, and flexibility, and the exercises on this page can all be done at home as you become 'fit for birth'.

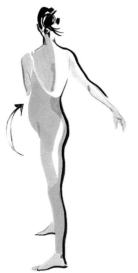

Waist and spine (mobilizes)
Left: Stand with feet slightly apart and arms relaxed. Without moving the hips, twist from the waist first to the right and then to the left, allowing your head to follow the movement. The spine should remain upright.

Hips (suppleness and flexibility)
Right: Practise this position whenever you can, when reading or watching television, Sit with the feet together and the knees apart. Ideally keep the back is supported.

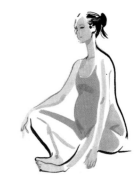

Stomach (strengthens)
Right: Lie on one side, with knees bent, and hands around abdomen. Breathe in deeply, then exhale, pulling in the stomach.

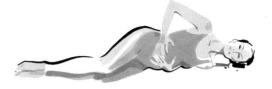

Spine (lengthens)
Right: Lie on your back with legs together and arms outstretched behind head. Breathe in deeply, and stretch further as you exhale.

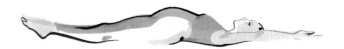

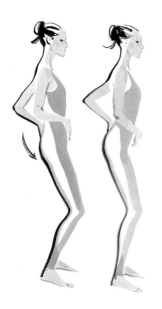

EXERCISE AFTER BIRTH

Just as the birth will be a very individual experience so the exercise you take afterwards will vary. It will depend on what has happened to the abdominal muscles during pregnancy, whether it is your first or your fourth baby and the weight of the baby. After a natural birth, under guidance from your health visitor, you can start exercising within four to six weeks. If you have had a caesarean section however the abdominal muscles are very sensitive so you may have to wait a little longer.

The aim of exercising after birth is to make contact with your body in order to tone and strengthen it back to its pre-pregnant state. As well as the general exercises featured on this page remember to exercise your pelvic floor muscles using the techniques on page 43, since these are the muscles which will have probably undergone the most strain.

Lower back (loosens)

Above: Stand with feet slightly apart, knees bent, with one hand on the abdomen and the other on the lower back. Tilt the pelvis forward, tucking under the bottom, and then back. Keep a strong stomach throughout.

Stomach

Below: Sit upright with knees bent up and feet together, arms crossed in front of the chest. Breathe out tilting the pelvis forward, pulling the stomach in and leaning back slightly. Hold, then breathe in as you return to sitting upright.

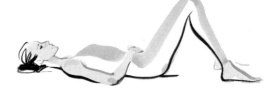

Abdomen (strengthens)

Above: Lie on your back with knees bent, feet hip width's apart, and hands resting on abdomen. Breathe in, and as you breathe out pull the abdomen in gently and tilt the pelvis upward. Hold, then relax.

Lower back (stretches)

Below: Lie on your back holding the knees. Breathe out, pulling in the stomach, and pull the knees towards the chest, Breathe in and relax.

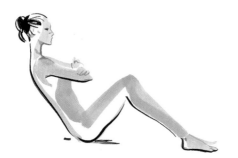

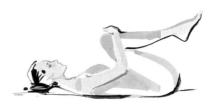

Arthritis and exercise

Arthritis is one of the most common diseases, affecting nearly a billion people worldwide. Its origins are still completely unknown, but it is not contagious and, unlike cancer or heart disease, it is rarely a direct cause of death. However, it can be completely disabling if you allow it to take over your life. Don't let it control you: it is possible to lead a full and active life despite arthritis, and exercise can play a major part in this.

Keeping your joints flexible and mobile will help to preserve their functioning as it assists the secretion of sinovial fluid (the lubrication need for joint movement) around the joint capsule. The Arthritis Association in the UK and the Arthritis Foundation in the USA both currently approve range-of-motion, muscle-strengthening and aerobic exercises, so long as each regime is individually tailored and is coupled with appropriate rest. However until recently the traditional exercise programme for arthritis was built purely around range-of-motion exercises interspersed with lots of rest. If the patient complained about weakness or fatigue they were advised to reduce their exercise. Although it is true that appropriate rest will help to reduce joint inflammation, it is now thought that excessive rest could actually be detrimental to health. Research has shown that in just one week of immobilization muscle can loose 30 per cent of its bulk. Such muscle weakness from lack of physical activity is very common in people with arthritis so by regaining muscular strength increased functional capacity and lessened disability is also achieved.

Exercise will also help to relieve some of the physical discomfort which accompanies arthritis. The pain may be worse first thing in the morning or after a period of rest, possibly because fluid leaks out of the blood vessels and lymph channels during sleep, flooding the tissues surrounding the joints. Exercise pumps the fluid out, back into the blood vessels and lymph channels, so cleaning the joints and reducing pain.

The other area in which exercise, although not a panacea,

BENEFITS OF EXERCISE

For those patients suffering from arthritis, a carefully monitored exercise programme can help prevent immobility in the musculo-skeletal system and so reduce the risk of:
• Weakness and hence wasting of muscles, ligaments, tendons and bones.
• Joint cartilage degeneration.
• Osteoporosis and subsequent bone fracture.
• Shortening of muscles, tendons, ligaments and joint capsules, which limits the range of a joint's motion and impairs mobility.

can have profoundly beneficial effects is the psychological problems associated with arthritis. When you discover that you have a chronic disease, the emotional pain and great loss of self-esteem can be more disheartening than the physcial pain. There can be immediate worries about the future and changes in lifestyle that at the time can seem almost unbearable.

However, studies have found that people who exercise on a regular basis suffer substantially less stress, anxiety and depression in such circumstances and in addition can improve the quality of their sleep. Ken Cooper, of the Cooper Clinic in Dallas, Texas, likes to tout exercise as 'nature's own tranquillizer'. He and others believe that this tranquillizing effect occurs to some extent because exercise triggers the release of endorphins, the hormones produced by the pituitary gland. When they enter the bloodstream these endorphins relieve pain and bring about a sense of cheerfulness.

The aim when exercising should be to avoid the development of contractures, a shortening of the muscles. Keep the joints extended – that is, fully straightened out when you are sitting, standing or lying down. You can do this by putting your feet up when sitting in an arm chair, letting your arms drop at your sides when standing upright and not bending your arms or legs when lying flat.

In addition to the three types of exercise listed left the ideal exercise program will also include some resistance rubber-band exercises (see page 162). Start off gradually with a little of each and then slowly build up to a comfortable but not painful level. Do, however, consult your medical doctor before any exercise, since people who suffer from arthritis inevitably run the risk of doing the wrong kind, which could worsen their condition.

A good way to start exercising is with the fingers, as the hands are often the first to show signs of arthritis. The exercises on page 157 are all good for both stretching and mobilizing, but you can also try finger strengtheners which are available from Lyon Equipment Ltd (see page 219), or therapeutic putty and hand grips from most sports shops. These are all useful for arthritic conditions in hands.

WHICH TYPE OF EXERCISE

The three most important types of exercise for arthritis sufferers are:

• Range-of-motion and stretching exercises.

• Muscle-strengthening exercises which don't place excess stress on affected joints.

• Aerobic exercise such as swimming, brisk walking, cycling and dancing.

FINGER EXERCISES

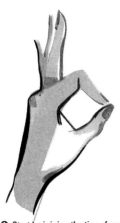 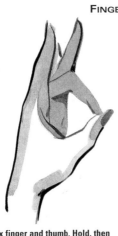 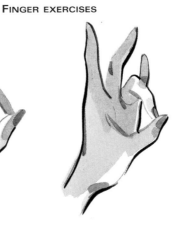 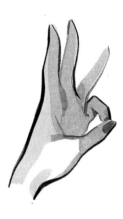

❶ Start by joining the tips of your index finger and thumb. Hold, then straighten your index finger and bring your middle finger to your thumb. keeping the other fingers as straight as possible.

❷ Continue with the other two fingers in turn and then repeat using the other hand. To strengthen the fingers as well, press the fingertips firmly together each time the thumb is joined by a finger.

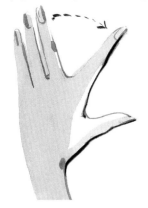 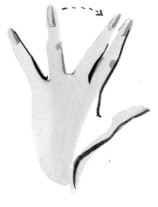

❶ *(Left hand shown)* Rest your hand on a flat surface, with the fingers together and the thumb outstretched. Slide the index finger towards the thumb, trying to keep the other fingers still. Then slide the other fingers across in turn.

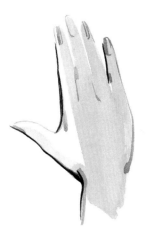 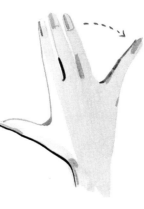

❷ *(Right hand shown)* Once all the fingers have moved across to the thumb, starting with the little finger, slide each back in turn away from the thumb. Again, when moving one, try to keep the other fingers still.

Exercising after a stroke

BENEFITS OF EXERCISE

A rehabilitation programme of exercise and physiotherapy within the first six months after a stroke can help:

• Reverse neurological malfunctions.

• Eliminate physical impairment such as paralysis and loss of sensation.

• Remedy mental confusion.

Continued moderate exercise for at least a year afterwards may:

• Reduce the extent of physical disability.

• Improve functional capacity.

• Lower high blood pressure, one of the most imprtant risk factors for a stroke.

• Reduce the chance of a second stroke.

WHICH TYPE OF EXERCISE

After a stroke patients should include all three forms of exercise in their programme:

• Range-of-motion and stretching.

• Muscle-strengthening.

• Aerobic exercise such as swimming, brisk walking, cycling and dancing.

No two strokes are ever the same. The various factors that influence recovery and after effects include the type of the stroke and the extent and location within the brain of its damage. As the neurological pathways are crossed, when the left side of the brain is partially damaged, it is the right side of the body which will be affected. The left side of the brain also controls speech and language and behaviour, so changes may occur in these areas. Right brain damage in contrast affects the left side of the body and may impair the ability to judge distance and speed of movement.

Stroke sufferers are normally started on a rehabilitation programme of moderate exercise, physiotherapy and relaxation therapy as soon as possible. This is carried out by a team of specially trained occupational, speech and physical therapists, nurses and social workers who work closely with the patient and often with a family member.

When the rehabilitation programme has finished, usually after a period of six months, many patients cease to exercise as they believe that their improvement has reached its limit. However continued exercise can bring further recovery.

A study conducted by physical therapists from Pacific University in Oregon evaluated changes in stroke patients who were at least one year removed from their strokes, over one month's intensive rehabilitation including physical exercise. Positive improvements were noted in their functional capacities and it was concluded that significant improvements could still be achieved at this late stage.

Having a stroke is like a recurrent disease, and continued exercise together with relaxation therapy may also help fight the causes of a stroke, such as high blood pressure, and thus reduce the likelihood of another. Exercise will not cure a patient from the damaging effects of a stroke, but if performed in consultation with a medical doctor, it is undoubtedly a highly effective supplementary therapy.

Methods of exercise

The methods of exercising described on the following pages represent only a handful that you may like to try, each with its own distinct advantages and disadvantages. The most important thing is that you choose a type of exercise you enjoy. Begin with five minutes a day and gradually build up over the weeks. And, of course, always consult your medical doctor before taking up any exercise if you are in any doubt about a particular health condition.

REBOUND EXERCISE

Rebound exercise is extremely simple and incredibly effective. A rebounder is a circular mini-trampoline with a padded edge which is used by just running or jumping on it. It is a very manageable way of increasing aerobic exercise in the privacy and convenience of your own home.

All exercises work on the basis of opposition to the gravitational pull of the earth. The increased gravitational pull from rebounding in particular strengthens the skeletal system which in a sedentary lifestyle is relatively weak. Studies of astronauts have found that after just two weeks in outer space exposed to decreased gravity they lose 15 percent of their bone mass and can thus suffer from osteoporosis.

The overall effect of rebounding is to provide a complete physiological cellular masage. As the cells are stressed and take in the oxygen necessary to 'burn' carbohydrates, fat or protein, they force waste products into the surrounding fluids. Through stimulation the cells become stronger and the extra-cellular fluid movement is increased.

Rebounding is also a great way of circulating the lymphatics (the body's internal cleansing system). As you bounce on a rebounder the valves in the system open at the top of the bounce while at the bottom the cells squeeze the toxins and waste out from around the cellular tissue spaces, thus allowing the cleansing lymph to flow up as the body starts to descend.

BENEFITS

Running on a trampoline jars much less than on the ground. Rebound exercise can be beneficial in the following ways. It can:

• Eliminate shock to the weight-bearing joints.

• Help prevent 'jogger's disease', a kidney condition indicated by an abnormal presence of protein, red blood cells and other substances in the urine.

• Strengthen the skeleton, so reducing the risk of osteoporosis.

• Increase cardiovascular activity and physical fitness by efficient circulation of oxygen, blood and body fluids.

• Keep the body healthy by circulating the lymphatics that open and close as you jump up and down.

• Improve weight loss by the burning of carbohydrates.

BENEFITS

The resistance band technique is
particularly beneficial for:

• Mobilizing joints.
• Increasing circulation to muscles
and joints.
• Strengthening major muscle groups.
• Improving posture.
• Helping reduce back problems by
strengthening the spinal musculature.
*As always check with your doctor
before embarking on the exercise if
you suffer from back or joint pain.*

THE RESISTANCE BAND METHOD

The resistance band method of exercising uses a specially
designed band approximately 10–15cm/4–6in wide made of
durable latex. The resistance band provides an even tension for
muscles to resist during various movements and is suitable for
all age groups and levels of fitness. It enables you to isolate
certain parts of the body and therefore avoid any areas likely to
cause problems.

With care, the resistance band can easily be used at home. It
is available from most sports shops and all you need in
addition is a floor mat or towel for the floor exercises. For safe,
comfortable exercising, it is advisable to dust the band before
use lightly with talcum powder. This, and using nothing tighter
than a loose knot or half-bow will enable you to tie and untie
the band easily. To prevent the band from digging into the
hands or sliding up the legs try to maintain the natural width of
the band as you exercise. Finally, men should remember to
wear socks high enough to prevent the band pulling at leg hair.

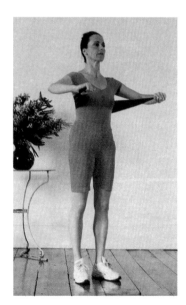

Upper chest and back muscles
❶ Stand with the band around the upper
back, and raise bent elbows. Breathe in.

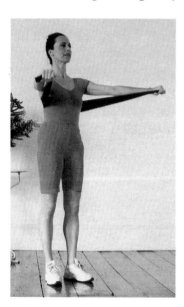

❷ As you extend the arms to the sides,
breathe out. Breathe in and return arms to the
bent elbows position. Repeat to other side.

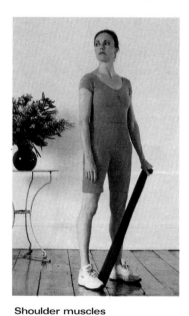

Shoulder muscles
❶ Place your right foot on one end of the
band and hold the other end in the left hand.

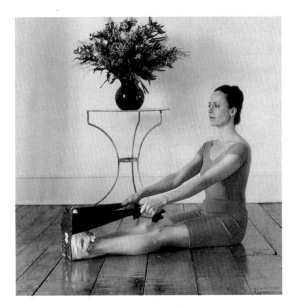

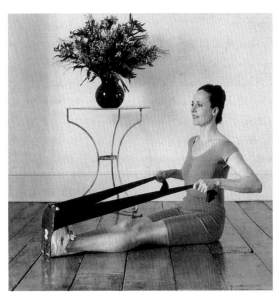

Upper back and shoulder muscles

❶ Sit on the floor with legs straight ahead and wrap the band round the ends of both feet. Hold the ends in outstretched arms.

❷ Pull the ends of the band in towards the chest, the back upright and the shoulders well down. Slowly return the arms to their outstretched position.

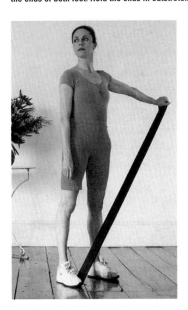

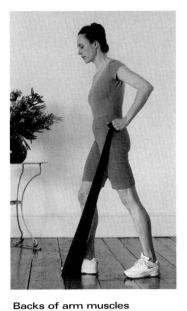

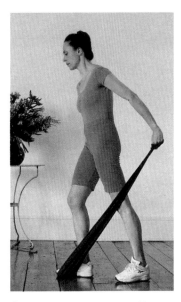

❷ With the elbow slightly bent, lift the left arm sideways up to shoulder level and then slowly lower again. Repeat to other side.

Backs of arm muscles

❶ Step forward with right foot onto one end of the band. Hold the other end in left hand.

❷ Without twisting the arm, extend it backwards, keeping the shoulders down, then slowly bend it back. Repeat to other side.

BENEFITS

The Lotte Berk technique is beneficial for:

• Stimulating the heart and glands.

• Increasing the flow of adrenaline.

• Ridding the body of accumulated toxins.

• Relieving back, neck and shoulder problems.

• Toning thighs, bottoms, stomachs and waistlines.

THE LOTTE BERK TECHNIQUE

The Lotte Berk Technique is a series of exercises designed to stretch and relax every muscle in the body. It was developed more than thirty years ago by Lotte Berk, an accomplished German dancer who was discovered by Dame Marie Rambert in the 1930s. Lotte was acclaimed as a great interpreter of modern dance and years later, when she gave up her dancing career, she began teaching exercise to women, using a technique for non-dancers devised from modern ballet.

It was during this teaching period that Lotte had a serious fall which caused extensive damage to her lumbar vertebrae. Thanks to the rigorous exercise programme she then followed she made a miraculous recovery and 14 days after the accident she was able to walk proudly back into her doctor's surgery.

Inspired by her success, Lotte then worked closely with an osteopath and with the addition of orthopaedic movements she devised her own unique exercise regime. Now in her mid-80s but looking years younger, Lotte still exercises regularly despite suffering from osteoporosis and, with a petite and wonderfully slim figure, she is the perfect advertisement for her own regime. She believes there is no need for any woman to lose her figure after childbirth or have an old and decrepit body in maturity – the list of other women who now practise her exercises is endless.

Based on modern ballet, yoga and orthopaedics, regular sessions of the exercises will help to tone bulging thighs, sagging bottoms, weak stomachs and shapeless waistlines. To begin with, it is advisable to attend the classes, but once you have mastered the exercises – there are 34 in total – you will be able to practise them at home. Three of her most popular exercises are illustrated opposite – the first will stretch and tone the legs and is to be performed both legs, the second will work both the legs and thighs and the third concentrates on strengthening the stomach. Those with weak stomach muscles, may like to practise this last exercise with their feet tucked under a bed or sofa for support.

Lotte Berk classes are available in various areas of London, Bath, Winchester, New York, Rome and Zurich. (see page 219).

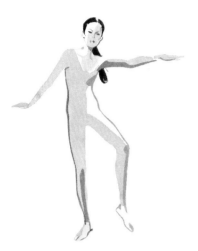

❶ Hold on to a chair, with left arm at shoulder level. Pointing the foot, raise the left leg diagonally in front and lean towards it.

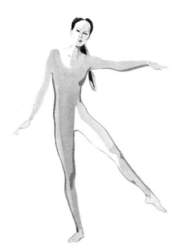

❷ Stretch the left leg, and point your toes, keeping the hip stationary.

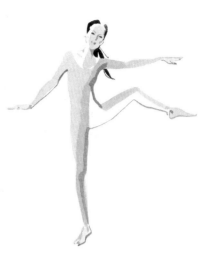

❸ Bend the knee again, and lift your leg higher, continuing out to a stretch. Repeat 3 times.

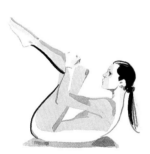

❶ Lie on your back and curl your body round, bringing knees and head together.

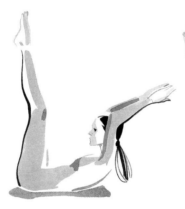

❷ Keeping your spine well into the floor, push legs upwards and lift arms back above the head.

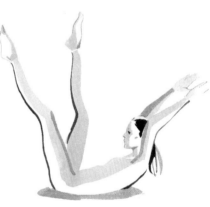

❸ Do a walking movement with the legs in the air, pull up with the diaphragm and stretch arms up high. Try for 10-20 walks.

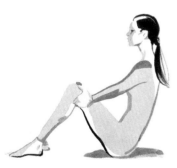

❶ Sit on the floor with knees bent, and hands holding thighs.

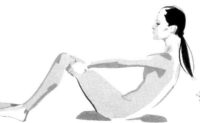

❷ Curl back down to the floor through the spine vertebrae, moving only the pelvic area.

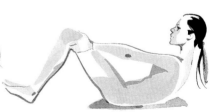

❸ Continue the movement as low as you can. Repeat 5 times.

BENEFITS

The Alexander technique has proven beneficial for sufferers of:

- Digestive problems.
- Heart and lung conditions.
- High blood pressure.
- Headaches.
- Sciatica.
- Arthritis.
- Backache.
- Neck and shoulder tension.
- Stress-related illnesses.
- Breathing disorders.

THE ALEXANDER TECHNIQUE

The Alexander Technique, founded by an Australian actor, Frederick Matthias Alexander, is a way of improving posture and physical control and enabling the body to work in a more relaxed and capable manner.

When the natural subconscious procedures for balance and posture are disturbed by injury or maltreatment, our mental and physical functioning can become adversely affected. This is due to the impairment of the body's automatic reflex responses which under normal circumstances when they are working correctly support the body. The Alexander Technique aims to prevent obstruction of these complex mechanisms and restore their efficacy.

The technique has helped people from all walks of life by improving their health and emotional wellbeing, and adding to their lives a new dimension of awareness and creativity. It addresses the underlying causes of many cases of back pain, neck and shoulder tension, stress-related illnesses and breathing disorders where improper posture is a contributory factor. Since spinal posture imbalance and the resulting curvature can also cause problems to the internal organs, it can also help digestive, heart and lung problems.

The lessons focus on the connections between thought and action and particularly the practical effects of thought on muscle activity. When instructed and channelled correctly, thought processes can help to release tension, allowing the body to become correctly aligned and the energy flow to be balanced. Many people, as their posture has improved and they have begun to stand completely upright again, have actually experienced the sensation and physical results of beoming taller thanks to the Alexander Technique.

Once you have learned the technique from a qualified teacher (see page 219 for where to find one) it can be applied anywhere, such as during work, at the office, at home, and during sports and leisure activities. It is particular popular amongst actors and performers on stage and for those who practise it natural poise and composure soon become a way of life.

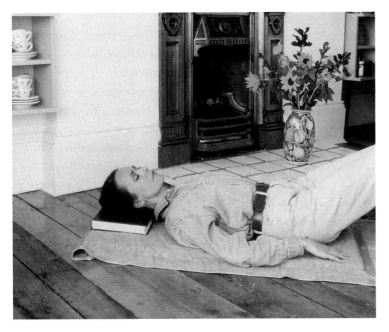

Relaxation position

Left: In order to align the spine, place a small book under the head and raise the head in line with the rest of the body. The hips should be absolutely level.

Incorrect posture

Below left: As far as possible avoid sitting with the shoulders rounded, the stomach out and legs or feet crossed.

Correct posture

Below right: Aim to sit with the back straight and well supported, shoulders down and legs relaxed and together.

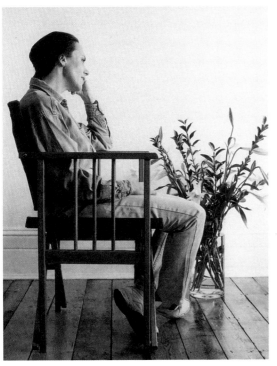
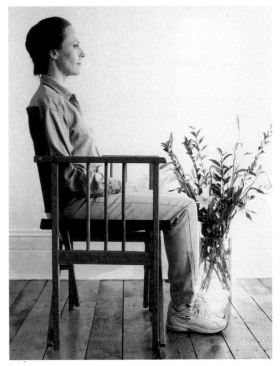

BENEFITS

Pilates can be beneficial in many ways. It can:

- **Restore flexibility and joint mobility to the young and elderly.**
- **Improve co-ordination, balance and alignment.**
- **Eliminate bad postural habits.**
- **Alleviate back pain.**
- **Prevent the onset of brittle bones.**
- **Help calm repetitive strain injury.**
- **Reduce stress.**
- **Create a greater resistance to disease by stimulating the circulation and immune systems.**
- **Tone slack muscles.**

PILATES

Pilates is a form of exercise which co-ordinates the working of the muscles with the breathing. It tones the whole body and improves posture by following a carefully developed method perfected over a period of more than 60 years of experience and observation. The crucial feature of Pilates in comparison with some other techniques is that it focuses completely on how you perform an exercise, and carry yourself in daily life. What you do is less important.

It was developed in the early 1920s by Joseph Hubertus Pilates, who was born in Dusseldorf in 1880. As a child he was very frail and anxieties over contracting tuberculosis prompted him to start body building. By the age of 14 he was posing for anatomy charts and studying them enthusiastically. In 1912 he decided to go to England, where he earned his living as a boxer, an instructor of self-defence and a circus performer. At the outbreak of war along with all other German residents in the country, he was detained in England and it was during this period that he fully developed his ideas about health and body building.

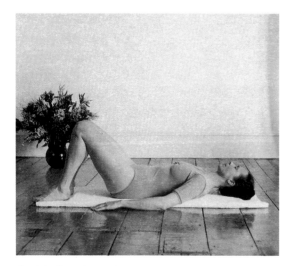

Lie on the floor, with feet slightly apart. Pull the navel towards the spine without altering the line of the hips. The spine should lengthen and relax into the floor.

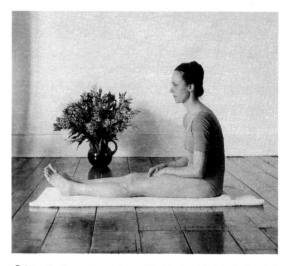

❶ Sit on the floor, with your legs outstretched, and feel the back curled over and the shoulders slightly hunched. This is how most people sit naturally, but it is an inefficient position which Pilates aims to improve.

After the war Pilates returned to Germany, where he was training the Hamburg police in self-defence when an invitation to train the new German army prompted him to leave for the USA. During the journey across he met Clara on the boat, whom he later married. Initially drawn to each other by their mutual interest in health, they then went on to open a physical fitness studio together in America. Joe and Clara worked at the Pilates studio for decades, but it was Joe who remained in charge of his method and continued to work with an endless energy well into his 80s.

The influence of Joe Pilates and his exercise method initially centred on the dance world in America but word eventually spread, and he created a following from people in many areas of society and business from films and theatre to music and medicine. Since the 1930s the Pilates method has grown in popularity and expanded tremendously. After America, the Europeans adopted it and nowadays there are studios all over the world. It is favoured as a 'cooling down' after any other form of exercise or sport. The technique can be performed in group classes with an instructor or using a Pilates machine.

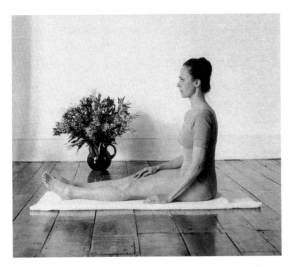

❷ Now, sit up out of the hips, and as if pulled up from the top of the head feel your back and neck lengthen and the shoulders gently relax down.

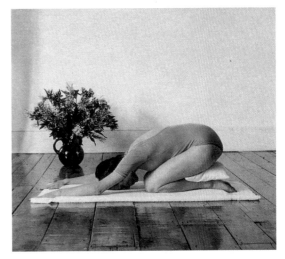

To relax and stretch the spine after back exercises, or for back ache, kneel on the floor with arms outstretched and keeping knees slightly apart and feet together, try to push the bottom down onto the heels.

PRINCIPLES OF PILATES

The pilates method is founded on the following eight principles:

- **Relaxation.**
- **Concentration.**
- **Co-ordination.**
- **Alignment.**
- **Centring.**
- **Flowing movements.**
- **Breathing.**
- **Stamina.**

How does it work?

Pilates works on the principle that control, centring, precision and correct breathing can result in an increase in body awareness, confidence and health. It proves that with a knowledge of exactly how the body works the shape of the body can be transformed, Pilates teaches you to become aware of the interrelations between the position and movement of each part of the body. For example, focusing your mind on 'centring' the area between the bottom of the rib cage and the top of the hip-bones can flatten the stomach and slim the waist. When using the muscles in this way it is important to be aware of working internally and not just peripherally.

Pilates is suitable for any age group and in conjunction with physiotherapy can benefit many problems such as back weaknesses or injuries, and knee problems, With a few adjustments to the standard programme and after consultation with a medical doctor, sufferers from high blood pressure can exercise safely using the Pilates method. It is also suitable for pregnant women, although there are certain modifications to be made for each stage of pregnancy. As with any exercise during these nine months the expectant mother's doctor should be notified in advance.

Pilates is easy to learn, but application can be more difficult as every individual's shape and metabolism varies. In addition each movement is accompanied by specific breathing techniques which when correctly co-ordinated will result in increased oxygenation and detoxification. A Pilates session is individually devised according to your posture and its needs for improvement and strengthening. It is taught on a one-to-one basis, and once the exercises are mastered it is possible to do many of the floor exercises on a mat at home.

Pilates can be used in conjunction with any other form of exercise as it balances the body. Swimming in particular complements Pilates, but care should be taken in cases of back and neck problems. Pilates teaches that the spine should always be kept as straight as possible, and some strokes, such as breast stroke done with the head lifted out of the water can place a strain on the back of the neck and cause the lower back to arch.

In helping to develop a new balance, both physically and mentally, few methods have emerged as successful as Pilates – as Joseph Pilates was fond of saying, quoting the famous German poet Friedrich von Schiller 'It is the mind itself which builds the body.'

For where to obtain further details on Pilates and information of classes in your area see page 219.

T'AI CHI

T'ai chi, meaning wholeness, is based on the belief that illness due to emotional disturbance usually arises from an imbalance in the flow of energy (known as Qi) either because it collects in one particular area or because it moves too fast or too slowly throughout the body.

Originating in China, t'ai chi has been practised now for many years in the west and ideally should take place in the open air. In addition to correcting the imbalance of energy throughout the body it aims to help people to focus on their mental and emotional state. It is based on a series of slow-moving graceful exercises which the Chinese consider to be beneficial for anxiety and stress. Its flowing movements can also help improve breathing, stimulate circulation and generally improve posture.

T'ai chi should be learned from a fully qualified teacher (see page 219
) as personal guidance is important for maintaining correct body alignment. Details of classes and courses can usually be found at your local library, leisure centre or health-food shops, as well as in magazines. The classes should be attended regularly as there are over 100 different movements to be learned – one or two classes a week would be ideal. Learning t'ai chi should not be rushed as there should be an emotional awareness with each individual movement. It is a wonderfully tranquil way of moving, encouraging body awareness and

BENEFITS

T'ai chi, if practised consistently, will:
- Improve breathing.
- Stimulate circulation.
- Realign posture.
- Alleviate stress and anxiety.
- Encourage a positive self-image.

Brain fitness

STIMULATING THE BRAIN

LEFT SIDE

The following activities will encourage the development of the left side of the brain concerned with logical thinking:

• Playing bridge.
• Playing chess.
• Filling in crosswords.
• Learning a language.

RIGHT SIDE

These activities are more appropriate for stimulating the right side of the brain concerned with creativity:

• Sewing.
• Painting.
• Calligraphy.
• Designing.

The human brain is the most incredible living organ ever created, yet it is still susceptible to the same life changes as the body. We are born with billions of brain cells, or neurons, but with time they begin to die and their efficiency gradually declines. In addition we start to lose the neurotransmitters or chemical messengers which transport information to and from nerve cells. The effectiveness of these messengers depends on how stimulated the ageing brain of an individual remains.

Professor Arthur Shimamura of the University of California, Berkley, USA, identifies three main ways in which mental function changes with age. The first is a lessening of mental speed as the efficiency of the brain's neurons reduces. Messages take longer to travel from the brain to the body, so an individual's reaction speed decreases in circumstances such as road traffic incidents.

The second way in which mental functioning changes is in the reduction in learning capacity. The temporal lobes (the area of the brain which controls new learning) become particularly vulnerable to the effects of ageing making it more difficult to master new technology and routines. As a result we have to rely on diaries and mental aids more.

The third brain system which weakens with age is the 'working memory', or mental notebook, which enables us to juggle our thoughts constantly and organize the day-to-day events of life. The working memory system is located in the frontal lobes of the brain, behind the forehead and above the eyes. This area of the brain is more vulnerable to the ageing process than any other part.

As we grow older, it is not so much that we lose our memory but that we accumulate more information to store, while at the same time our capacity to store it decreases. To remain mentally young we must exercise the mind as well as the body, and as a result we may give ourselves the opportunity to become yet more knowledgeable with age.

HOW TO IMPROVE YOUR MEMORY

We all yearn for a better memory and one of the ways to help encourage this is by increasing our general brain fitness. Just by working towards including some of the following ideas into your daily routine you can record substantial improvements.

• Maintain a good posture to assist bloodflow to the brain.

• Practise relaxation techniques for memory improvement. They can aid both speed and retention.

• Make lists or use 'post it' notes for things you need to remember.

• If you are constantly losing particular items such as your sunglasses or your watch, make sure that you create a special place for them where you know you will always be able to locate them.

• Reduce your consumption of alcohol as in the long-term it can dull the senses and reduce the brain's ability to store and process information.

• Stay off caffeine. According to Douglas Herman, author of Super Memory, caffeine is a proven memory killer. It also keeps you awake at night, which deprives you of the time needed to recharge the mind.

• Try ginko biloba,a herbal supplement, which can help the peripheral circulation and improve bloodflow to the brain.

• Try tyrosine, an amino acid which may also help as it is a precursor of dopamine, a kind of neurotransmitter.

EXERCISES FOR THE MENTAL MUSCLES

Here are a few suggestions for ways of increasing and improving your mental alertness.The best time to practise them is in the morning. Never do them last thing at night as they may keep you awake.

• Count out loud every alternate 'odd' number backwards from 100 as fast as possible.

• Recite the alphabet backwards as quickly as possible.

• Name out loud very quickly 20 different types of flower.

• Name out loud as quickly as possible 30 different objects beginning with the letter 'P'.

• Recite the seven times table as numbers only – 7, 14, 21, 28, 35 and so on.

• Try to remember, then say out loud the names of the ten last people you spoke to or saw. This could include personal and telephone conversations or, if you see few people, you could name ten people you saw on television, heard on the radio or read about in the newspaper.

• For 5–10 minutes a day hold a newspaper, book or magazine upside down in front of your eyes in a well lit area and read the words. The object is not so much to read quickly as this is an exercise geared towards stretching the brain rather than speeding the memory. To start with it will be a struggle and your reading speed will probably slow down as your brain tries to 'adapt' to the images and correct the words. It does get easier with practise.

Exercising the face

FACE IT

To maximise the benefits of exercise and to keep good facial tone and complexion:

• Moisturize regularly morning and night.

• Drink lots of water.

• Give up smoking.

• Eat a diet high in antioxidants (the vitamins A, C and E, and the mineral selenium).

• Don't stay too long in the sun.

• Maintain a regular weight.

There are nearly 60 muscles in the face alone and, like the muscles of the body, they will lose their shape if neglected. Throughout this chapter we have focused on the essentials of exercising the body and the mind, but it is equally important that we learn to exercise the face. After all, it is the most visible part of our bodies and the first to reveal signs of ageing and the effects of gravity.

As we grow older we lose the collagen and elastin which normally supplies us with elasticity and flexibility. The subcutaneous fat which lies just under the skin also diminishes, leading to 'sagging' of the skin. The result of this sagging skin is the appearance around the eyes of bags and hoods, and the jowls and neck becoming 'loose'.

Additionally, there is the age-old worry of wrinkles. Nowadays, bombarded with advertising women tend to think that daily applications of one of the many 'scientifically proven' anti-wrinkle creams on the market will give them their elixir of facial youth. We do not expect just by applying a cream to our thighs or buttocks we will combat fat or wrinkles in that area – exercise is the real key. The same applies to the face and we must exercise these muscles too to keep it toned and firm.

Your face is a mirror of your thoughts and emotions. Worrying can produce deep furrows in the forehead, sadness is often manifested by a 'downturned' mouth and even squinting can cause lines around the eyes. The muscles around the eyes are related to the nervous system and therefore worry, strain and lack of sleep are especially visible in this area of delicate skin.

The bone structure of the skull will largely dictate the shape of your face, but the layers of facial muscles can be changed through exercise. Facial exercise will also increase the skin's circulation, which will in turn improve the complexion and even help to reduce spots and enlarged pores. Remember, wrinkles do not have to be an inevitable part of ageing.

EXERCISES FOR THE FACE

Once you have mastered these exercises in front of a mirror, they can easily be incorporated into your day, when driving perhaps, or watching television. Massage the face gently with your fingertips in the direction of the arrows to intensify the results and boost circulation.

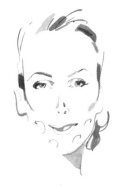

To firm the mouth

Left: To firm the mouth, roll the lips inwards over the upper and lower teeth, keeping the mouth slightly open. From this position, try to smile as wide as you can pushing outwards with your lower jaw.

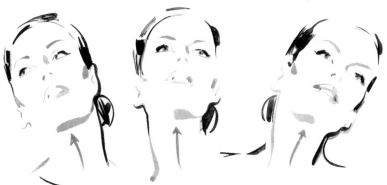

To firm the neck

Left: First curl the tongue towards the back of the mouth. Lift the chin, stretching up, and stretch your neck as far as possible to the right. Slowly rotate the head to the left, feeling the pull along the neck as you rotate it.

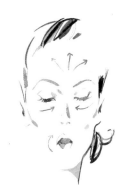

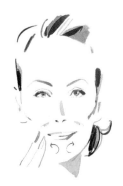

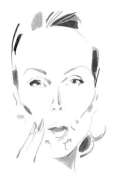

To tighten up skin on the face

Above: Make an 'O' shape with the mouth, pulling the upper lip down over the teeth. Shut your eyes and try to smile using the upper cheek muscles.

To smooth the upper lip and strengthen the mouth

Above: **❶** Keeping the eyes open, press and squeeze the lips tightly together, smiling slightly.

Above: **❷** Now pucker the lips to make a small 'O' and try to smile very slightly. Both stages of this exercise are particularly effective if used in conjunction with massage.

nutrition &
diet

NUTRITION & DIET

- Carbohydrates
- Proteins
- Essential fatty acids
- Vitamins
- Minerals
- Water
- Food allergy and intolerance
- Nutritional accessories
- Herbs

NUTRITION & DIET

Good nutrition should provide the body with the nourishment it needs. As we are all biochemically different, to maintain peak nutrition each of us has unique requirements.

Not many of us realize what it is like to feel really well as opposed to just not feeling ill. We often feel less than perfect – suffering from poor skin, muscle aches, indigestion, constipation, bags under or dark circles around the eyes, sinus problems and fatigue. We begin to accept these problems and feeling below par as normal, and often we are totally unaware of the reasons for feeling the way we do. The answer is usually that we are putting our bodies under too much strain by eating the wrong foods, smoking, drinking alcohol or not getting enough sleep.

Eating habits are formed early in life and can sometimes be difficult to change, but by looking closely at the balance of your diet you will be able to decide on a nutritional regime which will increase your health, energy and wellbeing. There is no need to go into complete denial, though. Have that special treat occasionally once you have acquired the correct balance – your body will soon tell you if you have overstepped the mark.

Avoid using food as an emotional prop. Eating starts in the mind, and if you are feeling down or angry, it is easy to use it for comfort, but then follows a feeling of guilt which takes you back to square one. Eat to nourish your body, not your fears.

The body requires vital nutrients: carbohydrates, proteins, essential fatty acids, vitamins, minerals, water and oxygen.

CARBOHYDRATES

Carbohydrates are converted by the body into glucose and glycogen and it is the digestion of carbohydrates which maintains the correct balance of blood sugar. About 75 per cent of the living world and about 75 per cent of the world's total calorie intake is made up of carbohydrates.

There are three types of carbohydrate: sugar, a simple carbohydrate; starch and fibre, both complex carbohydrates. Complex carbohydrates take more time to break down thereby entering the blood stream at a slower rate. The diet should contain about 50 per cent of complex carbohydrate, which is necessary for athletes for energy.

Unfortunately, for a quick 'boost' people snack on simple carbohydrates which are loaded with sugar and swiftly absorbed by the body. This raises blood sugar levels instantly and the body compensates by producing insulin. However, if this pattern is repeated over and over, the insulin levels remain high. As insulin is a major anabolic hormone this will result in the laying down of fat. The result is often visible as 'pot belly' in men and 'pear shape' in women and is compounded as we age by hormonal changes and a less active lifestyle. Complex carbohydrates are healthier for us simply because they are more slowly absorbed than simple carbohydrates and therefore the insulin 'highs and lows' are avoided.

PROTEINS

Proteins are essential for growth, general body repair and maintenance, and the production of enzymes which promote digestion, create hormones and produce antibodies to fight against infection.

The building blocks of proteins are known as amino acids and contain carbon, hydrogen, oxygen and nitrogen, all necessary for life. The main eight amino acids are:

Isoleucine Required for optimal growth and intelligence and used to synthesize other non-essential amino acids.

Leucine Stimulates brain function and increases muscular energy levels.

Lysine The building block of blood antibodies, strengthens the circulatory system and maintains normal growth of cells.

Methionine Maintains liver health, calms the nerves and is an anti-stress factor.

Phenylananine Required by the thyroid gland for the production of thyroxin for metabolic rate stimulation.

Threonine Improves intestinal incompetence and digestive assimilation.

Valine Stimulates mental capacity and muscle co-ordination.

SOURCES

Sources of complex carbohydrates include:
- Bread.
- Potatoes.
- Rice.
- Wholegrains.

Sources of simple carbohydrates include:
- Chocolate.
- Sweets.
- Cereal bars.
- Cakes.

SOURCES

Sources of proteins include:
- Poultry.
- Meat.
- Fish.
- Eggs.
- Dairy products.
- Soya beans.
- Seeds.
- Nuts and pulses.

Tryptophane Increases the utilization of the B vitamins, improves nerve health and the stability of the emotions.

All the essential amino acids are supplied in animal foods and they strengthen the natural metabolic reaction in our bodies.

Ideally our protein intake should be between 30 and 80g/1 and 2¾ oz daily of complete protein from animal foods. Plant foods do not always supply all the essential amino acids and are sometimes referred to as incomplete proteins. Excess protein, however, puts a strain on the digestive system and may in turn cause headaches, arthritis and mucus problems.

Vegetarians and vegans sometimes lack protein, and for these people protein powder drinks, many of which are dairy-free, are suitable. Amino acid supplements are also available.

COMBINING PROTEINS & CARBOHYDRATES

Proteins and carbohydrates need different digestive conditions. Proteins need an acidic environment and carbohydrates an alkaline one. However, if the stomach is not producing enough acid for protein digestion and the intestines are not alkaline enough, these foods can literally 'fight' as neither will have been properly digested. All starch foods should be thoroughly chewed otherwise the small intestine, though alkaline, is unable to complete what the pytalin (an enzyme in the saliva) began higher up in the digestive tract.

In the early 1900s an American, Dr William Hay devised a diet to combat such problems of digestion. He also stressed the importance of ensuring a chemical balance in the diet by consuming food with the correct acid and alkaline content. In our excretions the alkaline loss is four times greater than the acid loss, so it is the alkaline we need to replace. The ideal diet should contain 70–80 per cent alkaline-forming foods and 20–30 per cent acid-forming foods. An overly acid diet leads to a wide number of digestive and inflammatory conditions.

Many people find the Hay diet beneficial, simply because they are including more fruit and vegetables in their diet than they would normally and, as a result their digestion, absorption and energy levels improve, giving them a better quality of life.

RULES OF THE HAY DIET

• Starches and sugars should not be eaten with proteins and acid fruits at the same meal.

• Vegetables, salads and fruit should form the main part of the diet.

• Proteins, carbohydrates and fats should be eaten in small amounts.

• Refined and processed foods should be avoided.

• An interval of around four hours should elapse between meals of different food types.

FATS

Fat is extremely important for our health provided it is of the right type. Naturally occurring fat is not the enemy in a modern-day diet. The main problem is too much of the wrong kind and not enough of the right kind.

All fats and oils contain different fatty acids which affect the body in various ways. These fatty acids consist of carbon, hydrogen and oxygen in varying proportions. The fats and oils are categorized into saturated and unsaturated fats; the latter subdivide into monounsaturates and polyunsaturates.

The fats which occur in our diet

Saturated fats Contain the maximum amount of hydrogen. Butter, cheese, eggs, fatty meat and lard contain a large amount of saturates. These are now commonly thought to be the 'enemy' especially in terms of heart disease.

Monosaturated fats Contain less hydrogen than saturated fat. The main sources are olive oil, rapeseed oil, fruit, nuts, avocados and seeds.

Polyunsaturated fats Have the least amount of hydrogen and are found in oily fish, fish oils and most vegetables, which contain the essential fatty acids from which the omega-6 and the omega-3 families originate. These are beneficial for high blood pressure, dry skin, arthritis, water retention, impaired sight and memory loss.

Trans fatty acids These are damaged polyunsaturated fats. They can be created by the process of hydrogenation and some are industrially hardened to avoid rancidity. Trans fatty acids can increase blood cholesterol and are found in processed foods such as cakes, biscuits, crisps and pies.

The omega-6 family Omega-6 is derived from linolenic acid and is converted into gamma-linolenic acid (GLA) by the body. Its conversion depends on vitamin B6, magnesium, zinc and biotin which assists the necessary enzyme needed. The richest sources of GLA are evening primrose oil and borage oil; it is also found in sunflower, sesame, walnut, pumpkin, corn, olive, soya bean and wheatgerm oils or seeds. GLA is eventually converted into a hormone like substance called prostaglandin type 1 which has numerous benefits: it can relax blood vessels, lower blood pressure, maintain water balance throughout the body, assist insulin in balancing blood sugar levels, reduce pain and inflammation, thin the blood and improve immune functioning. A deficiency in omega-6 may occur in people with high blood pressure, PMT or breast pain, dry skin or eczema, inflammatory problems and MS, and in heavy drinkers.

The omega-3 family Omega-3 is derived from linolenic acid which is converted into EPA (eicosapentaenoic acid) and DHA (docosahexaenoic acid) from which prostaglandin type 3 is made. This prostaglandin is essential for correct brain functioning and muscular co-ordination, controlling cholesterol, improving metabolism, vision and learning ability. It also improves immune functioning, reduces inflammation, thins the blood and maintains water balance. The best sources are flax (linseed) oils, pumpkin, soya bean and rapeseed oils, and oily fish such as salmon, sardines and mackerel.

REDUCING YOUR FAT

To cut down on fat, try the following:

• Use skimmed or semi-skimmed milk.

• Substitute cream with low-fat fromage frais or low-fat yoghurt.

• Always remove skin from chicken.

• Bake potatoes instead of frying them. Beware the high-fat knob of butter!

• Steam, grill or boil food.

• Use polyunsaturated low-fat spreads instead of margarines, spread thinly.

• Substitute high-fat cheeses with cottage cheese.

• Use liquid cold-pressed vegetable oils such as sunflower, safflower, olive and rapeseed instead of hard fats.

• Check food labels carefully for the fat content.

How much fat should we eat?

The Department of Health in Britain has suggested that fats should provide around 35 per cent of the total daily calorie intake. Health experts have recommended 30 per cent and some even less, around 20 per cent. A 20 per cent intake should be composed of around 7.5 per cent polyunsaturates (which include omega-6 and omega-3), 7 per cent monounsaturates and 6 per cent of saturates.

The average fat intake in countries eating a western diet is estimated at 40 per cent or more, whereas countries like Japan, the Philippines and Thailand consume only about 15 per cent of total calorie intake as fat and consequently have a low incidence of fat-related diseases.

A certain amount of fat is needed to stimulate the production of bile. Without enough fat too little bile is formed, which prevents the gallbladder from emptying properly. This could then contribute to the formation of gallstones. Fat is also vital for the absorption of the fat-soluble vitamins such as A, D, E and K. These vitamins cannot be transported through the intestinal wall into the blood without the presence of fat. Remember that children need essential fatty acids for their development and healthy growth. All fats are fattening, so to reduce your waistline without reducing your health, cut down on fats in your own diet – don't cut them out altogether.

VITAMINS & MINERALS

Vitamins and minerals are naturally occurring substances which provide the body with essentials for life. In an ideal world we should obtain all the necessary vitamins and minerals from the foods we eat, but unfortunately during this century the planet has changed dramatically. A continuously growing population has generated the development of factory farming and artificially fertilized soil which has now lost many of its trace minerals. These, coupled with the growth of pollution and the consumption of processed foods, mean that our diet is often deficient in important nutrients.

By improving the diet and supplementing it when necessary we can improve body maintenance, combat stress and pollution and regenerate good health. It is never too late to heal the body even if it has been neglected in the past.

There are 13 major vitamins, most of which the body is unable to manufacture itself. These are divided into two groups. The fat-soluble vitamins, A, D, E and K, which dissolve in body fat and can be stored by the body. As they are not excreted in the urine excess intake should be avoided. The water-soluble vitamins, which include all the B group and vitamin C, dissolve in water. With the exception of vitamin B12 these cannot be stored in the body, which is why we need a regular supply of them.

Minerals are divided into two groups: macrominerals, which are required in fairly large amounts; and microminerals, which are needed in much smaller amounts. If the body's mineral intake becomes low, it draws from supplies stored in the muscles, liver and bones.

On the following pages are simple guides to vitamins and minerals to explain their individual properties.

RETAINING VITAMINS & MINERALS IN FOODS

Too often the natural vitamins and minerals available from food can be destroyed before they reach your plate. Here are a few tips to prevent loss of nutrients:

• Always buy fruit and vegetables as fresh as possible. Wash them well before eating, but don't leave them to soak for too long. Buy produce from your own country wherever possible as the vitamin content is often reduced during long journeys across the world.

• Try not to store fresh fruit and vegetables for too long and always keep them in a cool, dry, dark place.

• Eating raw fruit and vegetables is the healthiest way, but if cooking it is better to steam or microwave as boiling often destroys water-soluble vitamins such as B and C. This also applies to fish and rice.

• Once food is cooked eat it immediately. Keeping food hot or warming it up later destroys the vitamin C content.

• Freezing fresh produce is fine so long as when it is eventually cooked it is cooked thoroughly.

A SIMPLE GUIDE TO MINERALS

BORON A trace element important for calcium uptake.
Food source Leafy green vegetables, nuts, pulses, peas, grapes, apples, prunes and soya beans.
Functions Helps to synthesize oestrogen and vitamin D and reduce urinary excretion of calcium and magnesium. May be useful in arthritic and osteoporotic conditions and is currently being studied as an alternative to HRT.
Symptoms of deficiency Poor calcium absorption.

CALCIUM A macromineral. There is more calcium than any other mineral in the body.
Food source Milk and dairy products, tinned sardines and salmon (the bones are a good source of calcium), green vegetables, blackstrap molasses, tofu, soya beans, nuts, sunflower, sesame and pumpkin seeds.
Functions Builds and strengthens bones and teeth. Needed for all body functions. Calms the nervous system, aids sleep and maintains the correct pH balance of the blood. Important for vegans and vegetarians.
Symptoms of deficiency Osteomalacia, osteoporosis, back pain, muscle weakness, insomnia, cramps, rickets in children.

CHROMIUM A micromineral. An essential part of the glucose tolerance factor.

Food source Fish, shellfish, egg yolks, blackstrap molasses, red meat and liver, chicken, cheese, wholegrain cereals, fruit, nuts and grape juice.
Functions Regulates blood sugar and blood cholesterol levels, helps to transport amino acids to the liver and heart cells and lessens high blood pressure. Can also reduce sugar cravings.
Symptoms of deficiency Deficiency is uncommon but can be the cause of general weakness and fatigue.

COPPER A micromineral.
Food source Liver, most seafood, wholegrains, nuts, seeds, dried beans, almonds, apricots, walnuts, prunes and cocoa.
Functions Needed for bone growth and tissue formation, necessary for RNA, haemoglobin and iron absorption. Also helps to form melanin.
Symptoms of deficiency Increased risk of infection, hyperactivity and anaemia, but deficiency is unlikely in the west. *Too much copper can deplete zinc levels.*

IODINE A trace mineral mostly found in the thyroid gland.
Food source Seaweed, asparagus, watercress, seafood, garlic, eggs. Fruit and vegetables grown in iodine-rich soil.
Functions Essential for thyroxin formation and thyroid functioning, speeds metabolism and improves the condition of skin, hair and nails.

Symptoms of deficiency Coarse skin and hair, thyroid problems, slow metabolism.

IRON A micromineral.
Food source Liver, molasses, brewer's yeast, spinach, chickpeas, soya beans, meat, fish, wheatgerm, oatmeal, seaweed, leafy green vegetables and nuts.
Functions Essential for the formation of haemoglobin. Improves energy through the breakdown of proteins, carbohydrates and fats.
Symptoms of deficiency Anaemia, fatigue, headaches, reduced resistance to infection, insomnia and shortness of breath.
Vitamin C is important for iron absorption.

MAGNESIUM A macromineral.
Food source Fish, seafood, green vegetables, avocados, bananas, wholegrains, dried figs, pulses, nuts, soya beans, lentils, grapefruit, lemons and apples.
Functions Helps to utilize vitamins and other minerals, especially calcium. Reduces stress, assists nerve impulses and muscle contraction, regulates the body's acid/alkaline balance, maintains a healthy heart and is good for pre-menstrual tension.
Symptoms of deficiency Cramps and muscle tremors, blood sugar disorders, poor calcium deposition, insomnia, depression and fatigue.

MANGANESE A micromineral.
Food source Kidney beans, leafy green vegetables including spinach and watercress, nuts, seeds, egg yolks, oatmeal, organ meats and wholegrains.
Functions Helps enzymes generate energy and form bone and connective tissue, utilizes vitamins B, C and E, nourishes the brain and nerves, is good for tendon and ligament problems.
Symptoms of deficiency Poor muscle co-ordination and blood sugar disorders.

MOLYBDENUM A macromineral.
An essential component of a number of very important enzymes.
Food source Organ meats, wholegrains, dark leafy green vegetables, yeast and pulses.
Functions May prevent tooth decay and anaemia. Assists the production of DNA and RNA. Also believed to increase sexual potency in older men.
Symptoms of deficiency Tooth decay and anaemia.

PHOSPHORUS A macromineral.
After calcium, the second most well supplied mineral in the body.
Food source Wholegrain cereals, brown rice, milk, cheese, red meat, fish, poultry, nuts, seeds, eggs and brewer's yeast.
Functions Essential for many of the body's metabolic processes, builds and maintains bones, teeth, nails, hair and nerves. Necessary for the absorption of many nutrients.

Symptoms of deficiency
Weakness of muscles, osteomalacia, rickets in children, but generally deficiency is rare.

POTASSIUM A macromineral.
Food source Bananas, avocados, dried and fresh fruits, seeds, nuts, pulses, vegetables, meat and poultry.
Functions Works alongside sodium to maintain normal fluid levels in the body and stimulates elimination via the kidneys. Balances sodium levels. Essential for nerve impulse transmission. Good for oedema. Maintains acid/alkaline balance and right blood pressure. Athletes and sportspeople lose potassium through sweat.
Symptoms of deficiency Muscle weakness, tingling hands and feet, low blood pressure, constipation and nervous disorders.

SELENIUM A micromineral.
Food source Meat, fish, dairy products, fish and shellfish, wholegrains, brown rice, soya flour, brewer's yeast, broccoli, tomatoes and onions. Quality in the vegetables and grains depends on the level of selenium in the soil.
Functions An important anti-oxidant, protecting all fat-soluble vitamins from oxidation. Assists liver functioning. Semen has a high selenium content, so it is important for male reproductive capacity. Protects the red blood cells and maintains a healthy

immune system through the white blood cells. Slows the ageing process through its action on the damaging free radicals. Selenium works in conjunction with the vitamins A, C and E.
Symptoms of deficiency Impaired resistance to infection, male infertility and signs of ageing.

SILICON A trace element.
Food source Leafy green vegetables, brown rice, alfalfa and sweet (green/red/yellow) peppers.
Functions Strengthens bones, teeth, skin and connective tissue, balances blood pressure, can inhibit osteoporosis.
Symptoms of deficiency Brittle bones.

ZINC A micromineral.
Food source Shellfish, sardines, brewer's yeast, vegetables, peanuts, wholemeal and rye bread, brown rice, eggs, cheese, meat and wheatgerm.
Functions Essential for RNA and DNA formation, assists pituitary and adrenal gland metabolism. Beneficial for the nervous system, helps stress and depression. Speeds up wound healing, helps to prevent prostate problems and is an important immune system nutrient.
Symptoms of deficiency Slow wound healing, decreased resistance to infection, male impotence, white spots may appear on the nails.

A SIMPLE GUIDE TO VITAMINS

VITAMIN A Fat soluble. From retinol in animal foods or beta-carotene in plant foods.
Food source Oily fish, liver, butter, eggs and cheese contain retinol. Carrots, watercress, broccoli and other dark green vegetables, apricots, cantaloupe melon, tomatoes, pumpkin and parsley contain beta-carotene.
Functions Maintains healthy skin and mucous membranes. Prevents premature ageing in skin and bones. Promotes healing of wounds and burns. Necessary in the formation of an eye pigment involved in night vision. Needed for cell growth and development and immune system health. Anti-oxidant.
Symptoms of deficiency Poor night vision, susceptibility to skin infections and respiratory disorders.

VITAMIN B COMPLEX Water-soluble. A group of the B vitamins which are essential for the health of the nervous system. Beneficial for the condition of hair, skin and eyes. Any individual B vitamin should be taken alongside a B complex supplement to ensure the correct balance is maintained.

VITAMIN B1 (THIAMIN)
Food source Leafy green vegetables, liver, wheatgerm, cheese, eggs, pork, brewer's yeast, fruit, nuts, pulses and kidneys.
Functions Involved in the metabolism of carbohydrates, fats and alcohol for energy. Essential for digestion through utilization of sugars and starches and their conversion into glucose.
Symptoms of deficiency Can lead to low thyroid activity and heart palpitations, depression, lack of concentration, memory loss and irritability. Severe deficiency of thiamin rare in the west.

VITAMIN B2 (RIBOFLAVIN)
Food source Chicken, fish, milk, cheese, wheatgerm, leafy green vegetables, almonds, and yoghurt.
Functions Essential for growth, reproduction, healthy skin and eyes, mucus membranes, and metabolizing fats, carbohydrates and proteins. Good for sore, itchy or bloodshot eyes and for cataracts. Needed for functioning of vitamins B3 and B6.
Symptoms of deficiency Cracks at the corners of the mouth, itching and scaling of facial and scalp skin. Dental problems and light sensitivity.

VITAMIN B3 (NIACIN)
Food source Avocados, prunes, dates, eggs, wheatgerm, yeast, liver, figs, fish, meat, poultry, wholewheat and potatoes.
Functions Maintains normal blood cholesterol levels, important to nervous and digestive systems and synthesis of hormones, can help to regulate blood sugar, is useful for PMT, tinnitus, migraine and headaches. Energizes cells and is needed in the formation of neurotransmitters.

Symptoms of deficiency Depression, anaemia and fatigue. *Avoid niacin supplements in cases of gout, liver disease, stomach ulcers, diabetes and glaucoma.*

VITAMIN B5 (PANTHOTHENIC ACID)
Food source All meat, dried fruit, nuts, blackstrap molasses, brewer's yeast, wheatgerm, leafy green vegetables and wholegrains.
Functions Essential to cholesterol, fat and red blood cell synthesis. Required for the natural release of cortisone by the adrenal glands, needed for the healing of arthritis, asthma and rheumatism. Reduces fatigue, depression and insomnia. Generally anti-stress.
Symptoms of deficiency None.

VITAMIN B6 (PYRIDOXINE)
Food source Eggs, milk, organ meat, wheatgerm, blackstrap molasses, bran, potatoes, green vegetables, fish, pulses, prunes, nuts, yeast extract and bananas.
Functions Regulates body fluids and reduces oedema (swelling). Regulates protein metabolism and energy production. Important for immune function, formation of red blood cells and nervous system health. Helps prevent morning sickness and PMT and to protect arteries from atherosclerosis.
Symptoms of deficiency Anaemia, allergies, elevated cholesterol, seborrhic dermatitis and cracks around the lips.

Excess vitamin B6 is not compatible with Levadopa, a Parkinson's disease medication, or phenytoin or phenobarbitone, both anti-convulsant medicines.

VITAMIN B12 (COBALMIN)

Food source Pork, kidney, liver, eggs, beef, cheese, milk, green algae, miso and seaweed.

Functions Needed for cell division and for making RNA, DNA and myelin (the sheath surrounding nerve fibres). Helps neurological disorders, anaemia and post-natal depression. Can be stored in the body and needs calcium for optimum absorption.

Symptoms of deficiency Weakness in the nervous system, pins and needles, loss of sensation, reduced reflex response, jerking of limbs, possible thyroid and menstrual problems.

BIOTIN

Food source Liver, fruits, nuts, beef, kidney, brown rice, peanut butter and yeast extracts.

Functions Can inhibit candida, protects the body when taking antibiotic or sulphur drugs. Important in the synthesis of fat and cholesterol. Essential to healthy nervous tissue and bone marrow. Good for hair growth. Needed for vitamin C synthesis.

Symptoms of deficiency Fatigue, depression, muscular pain, skin disorders and sleepiness.

FOLIC ACID A co-enzyme with vitamins B12 and C.

Food source Leafy green vegetables, liver, carrots, egg yolk, rye flour, wholewheat, apricots, beans, melon, pumpkins, avocados, pulses and wheatgerm.

Functions Necessary for growth and division of cells and the production of RNA and DNA, especially in the regulation of embryonic and foetal nerve cell development. Can prevent premature hair-greying. Aids the production of hydrochloric acid, essential for digestion. Can improve lactation.

Symptoms of deficiency Fatigue, depression, sleeplessness and irritability. If a mother is deficient during pregnancy, her baby can be at risk of spina bifida.

VITAMIN C Water-soluble. The most essential of all the vitamins. We are unable to synthesize or store vitamin C in the body, which is why we need daily intake in food. It plays an important part in many areas of body health.

Food source Citrus fruits, leafy green vegetables, potatoes, broccoli, tomatoes, blackcurrants, green peppers, rose hips and strawberries.

Functions Maintains collagen (the body's intercellular 'cement'), necessary for the connective tissue. Can prevent premature ageing, heart and circulatory problems and colds. Alleviates hayfever as it is a natural histamine. Has antibiotic properties and is therefore good for infections and gastro intestinal disorders. Helpful for all kinds of stress as the largest accumulation of vitamin C is in the adrenal glands. Aids the absorption of iron from plant foods and is beneficial for vegetarians.

Symptoms of deficiency Frequent infections, bleeding gums, swollen and painful joints, slow wound healing, nose bleeds, easy bruising, wrinkling of skin, fatigue, and depression. Necessary for smokers and users of the contraceptive pill.

Excess vitamin C could interfere with testing for diabetes. People with kidney stones should not take high doses of vitamin C.

ESTER C (ASCORBATE) A rather special type of vitamin C as it is both fat- and water-soluble. It can therefore supply vitamin C more quickly at both tissue level and circulatory level than ordinary vitamin C which is constantly eliminated from the body. Ester C has shown a waste factor of one-third of the amount of normal excreted vitamin C, The reason is that Ester C contains natural vitamin C metabolites which are biochemically identical to those created by the body to metabolise vitamin C. Two to four times as efficient as other forms of vitamin C, Ester C has been hailed as *the* discovery in vitamin C research for 40 years. It is available as a supplement, but is expensive.

BIOFLAVONOIDS These are part of the of the vitamin C complex and include rutin, quercetin, citrin and hesperidin.
Food source Blackcurrants, cherries, rose hips, tropical fruits, apricots, the pith of citrus fruits and buckwheat.
Functions Anti-inflammatory and anti-oxidant. Strengthens capillary walls which help to prevent varicose veins, thread veins and bleeding gums. Beneficial for oedema, eczema, psoriasis, hypertension and lung infection. Quercetin is sometimes found helpful for those suffering from hayfever and asthma.
Symptoms of deficiency Nose bleeds, gum bleeding and ulcers.

VITAMIN D (CALCIFEROL)

Fat-soluble. This is formed in the human skin tissue through the action of ultra-violet light.
Food source Oily fish such as sardines, salmon and tuna, fish liver oils, milk and dairy products.
Functions Needed to absorb calcium (and therefore particularly important to vegans who may have difficulty in maintaining an adequate calcium

level) and phosphorus, assists bone and tooth formation, important in the prevention of osteoporosis, essential to thyroid and parathyroid function, helps to prevent tooth decay.
Symptoms of deficiency Osteomalacia (softening of the bones) and rickets in children.

VITAMIN E (TOCOPHEROL)

Fat-soluble. Tocopherol comes from the Greek *tokos* (birth) and *phero* (to bear), and is known as the fertility vitamin.
Food source Dark green vegetables including broccoli, parsley, wheatgerm, sesame and sunflower seeds, eggs, nuts, unrefined vegetable and seed oils including olive, sunflower, safflower and soya.
Functions Neutralizes free radicals, prevents oxidation by free radicals of unsaturated fatty acids, hormones and vitamins A and C. Improves circulation and maintains cardiovascular health as it is a natural anti-coagulant. Beneficial to the reproductive organs and male and female infertility. Good for keeping the skin healthy and rejuvenated. Essential for athletes, and

dancers to protect against the harmful effects of oxidation from increased oxygen intake.
Symptoms of deficiency Reproductive problems, fatigue, muscle weakness, slow red blood cell production and haemolytic anaemia (a reduced level of haemoglobin in the blood).
If on anti-coagulant drugs, medical supervision of vitamin E supplementation is advisable.

VITAMIN K (PHYLLOQUINONE) Fat-soluble. Formed by natural bacteria in the intestines.

Food source Green vegetables, live yoghurt, fish liver oils, liver, egg yolks, cow's milk, tomatoes, kelp and alfalfa.
Function Assists calcium metabolism and may play an important role in the prevention of osteoporosis and fractures. Essential for normal blood clotting and correct liver functioning. Important for nerves, tissue and longevity.
Symptoms of deficiency Excessive bleeding, nose bleeds, coeliac disease, colitis and bruising easily.

TAKING SUPPLEMENTS

As regards dietary nutrients, requirements vary according to an individual's state of health, age and present circumstances. The needs of a pregnant woman will differ from those of an elderly woman or someone convalescing after an illness.

• Some nutrients can be toxic if taken in excess; too much of one may imbalance another.
• No single nutrient can improve health: only the multiple interaction between nutrients can be beneficial.
• Prolonged use of one nutrient may produce biological stress.

• Take note of the RNI (reference nutrient intake) or RDA (recommended daily allowance) printed on labels.
• Consult a fully qualified nutritionist for recommendations on the correct dosage and whether to take with meals or in between meals.

SPECIAL DIETARY NEEDS

Menopause Calcium, magnesium, evening primrose oil, royal jelly and vitamin B6 can all be helpful.

Pregnancy Folic acid, which plays a vital role in foetal development, calcium to protect teeth and bones and vitamins A, B, C and D are needed during pregnancy. Some women may need extra iron.

Breastfeeding As above, with selenium, copper, zinc and vitamin B12. Medical advice should always be sought during pregnancy and breastfeeding before taking dietary supplements.

The contraceptive pill There may be a need to increase the B complex. It is not advisable to take excess vitamin C at the same time as the mini pill since it may counteract its benefits.

Skin problems For psoriasis and eczema evening primrose oil or starflower (borage) oils are high sources of GLA which can reduce the itching often associated with these conditions. Fish oils contain high levels of EPA and DHA which have anti-inflammatory and anti-allergenic properties. Flax (linseed) oil contains omega-3 essential fatty acids required for healthy skin together with vitamins A, B complex and C and zinc.

Stimulants Heavy smokers and drinkers of alcohol, tea and coffee may need to supplement the diet as these stimulants inhibit the body's metabolism. Vitamins B and C should be increased in smokers and alcohol drinkers.

The elderly Poor diet can lead to a vitamin C deficiency and lack of sunlight can deplete vitamin D. Fish liver oils can be very beneficial for all joint problems.

VEGETARIANISM & VEGANISM

Vegetarianism is no longer considered a way of life for health freaks; in fact it is estimated that 2–6 per cent of the population are vegetarians and some sources suggest that within ten years this could increase to 20 per cent. Women seem to be more disposed to vegetarianism than men.

A meatless diet need not be a drawback to health, but it is certainly not a panacea for all ills. A true vegetarian does not eat meat or fish, but may eat other animal produce such as eggs, milk and cheese. A vegan does not eat any animal produce whatsoever, thereby relying solely on plant foods. A partial vegetarian, or pescatarian, omits meats from the diet but still eats fish.

According to Reed Mongels, RD, PhD a nutrition advisor to the Vegetarian Resource Group in Baltimore, USA, vegetarians are healthier than meat eaters as they consume less animal fat. They also seem to suffer less constipation, generally have lower blood pressure and many have less risk of developing diabetes.

Getting enough protein seems to be the major problem with vegetarianism, but most foods such as bread, potatoes, beans, pulses, rice, eggs, vegetables, cheese and milk provide enough protein. Even vegans can obtain a certain amount of dietary protein without the eggs, meat and cheese.

The deficiencies which occur most often are iron, calcium, zinc, vitamin B12 and, in vegans, vitamin D. There are various non-meat sources of all of these:

Iron can be obtained from beans, pulses, dark green leafy vegetables, nuts, egg yolk, dried fruits and wholemeal flour. Include a food source of vitamin C such as tomatoes or oranges at the same meal to enable iron to be properly absorbed.

Calcium is found in milk, dairy products (soya products such as milk, cheese and tofu), dark green leafy vegetables, seeds and nuts. Vegans need to increase their intake of beans and green vegetables to maintain adequate calcium levels, especially if the main part of their diet is made up of fibre-rich foods which can make calcium difficult for the body to absorb. Alternatively they should take a calcium supplement.

Zinc is obtained from brown rice, eggs, peas, wholemeal and rye breads, cheese, pumpkin seeds and most vegetables. There is sometimes a problem with the absorption of zinc due to the fibre in the diet, so adequate supplies of zinc-rich foods should be eaten. Alternatively a zinc supplement may help.

Vitamin B12 is found in milk, dairy products, soya milk, green algae, seaweed, miso and yeast extracts. Vegetarians will get plenty of B12 from these foods, but vegans should try to increase their intake of yeast extracts and green algae.

Vitamin D is obtainable by vegetarians only from milk and dairy products. This poses a problem for vegans as there are no foods containing vitamin D.

Some multi-vitamin/mineral supplements are available specifically for vegetarians and vegans, but get as many of the necessary substances from food sources as possible.

To become a vegetarian, change your eating habits gradually as the body, especially the metabolism, needs time to adapt. Beware of your intake of dairy products with a high fat content. Increasing fibre may cause abdominal bloating or flatulence initially, but eventually you will be able to combine as many ingredients as possible to ensure a good nutritional balance.

For further information contact the Vegetarian Society or Vegan Society (see page 219).

FIBRE

All plant foods provide dietary fibre. Fibre has very few calories, no nutritional value and provides little food energy to the body. However, although we are unable to digest or absorb it, the health of our digestive system benefits enormously from a regular intake of fibre. By adding bulk it helps the system to push waste products, cholesterol, bile acids and toxins right out. Fibre also nurtures bacteria in the large intestine.

There are two types of fibre: soluble (which dissolves in water) and insoluble (which does not). Soluble fibre, collects bile acids and other toxins while moving through the digestive tract, eventually removing them from the body. Cellulose and other components in insoluble fibre add bulk to the body's waste products, speeding their passage through the bowel.

Lack of fibre has been associated with a number of health problems, including constipation, diabetes (fibre helps to control blood sugar levels), high blood pressure, diseases of the large intestine, ulcers, varicose veins, weight gain, high cholesterol and breast cancer. Several studies have shown that a high-fibre diet reduces the risk of breast cancer. Researchers believe that excess oestrogen binds with wheat fibre and is eliminated in the faeces.

SOURCES

Good sources of soluble fibre include:

- Oats.
- Pulses.
- Wholemeal bread.
- Most fruits (including dried).
- Vegetables.

Insoluble fibre is mostly found in:

- Wholegrain bread.
- Bran.

WARNING

• Too much of one particular source of fibre can reduce iron and calcium absorption. It is advisable to include fibre from a variety of different foods.

• Always drink plenty of water otherwise the fibre could have a reverse effect and clog up the system.

THE IMPORTANCE OF WATER

Without water we would die. Existent in our cells and body tissues, it plays an essential role in nearly all our biological processes, including digestion, circulation and respiration. It lubricates our joints and eyes, regulates our body temperature, assists the elimination of toxins and waste products and transports nutrients around the body. Each day we lose about 300ml/½ pint of water through the simple act of breathing. Additionally we are losing water in our urine and perspiration.

Many people are in a permanent state of dehydration as a result not only of insufficient water consumption, but also of the diuretic effects of tea, coffee and alcohol. A diet of refined and processed foods, which is usually high in salt and sugar, is also dehydrating. These factors, combined with the effects of pollution and central heating, are literally drying us up. As we lose water, we also lose valuable electrolytes (essential minerals in water) such as sodium and potassium, which in turn causes us to feel mentally and physically below par. If we do not drink enough water, all sorts of problems can arise such as headaches, skin conditions, digestive problems, and kidney and bladder infections. Our sensitivity to thirst begins to diminish with age, which accounts for many elderly people being constantly dehydrated.

We obtain a certain amount of water from solid foods, fruit and vegetables having the highest content. For instance cucumbers and tomatoes consist of 93–96 per cent water. Melons also have a high water content, as do grapes.

First thing in the morning on wakening a common habit is to put the kettle on for coffee or tea when in fact what the body really needs is water as it has been deprived for hours during sleep. A glass of water on rising will replenish the system, whereas a cup of coffee will immediately dehydrate the system as it is diuretic.

Ideally you should drink 1½–2 litres/2½–3½ pints of water daily, not including the water in tea, coffee, fruit juices, soft drinks and herb teas. These drinks may quench your thirst initially, but they eventually sap the body of its fluids. Limit your intake of

foods high in sodium as they will also dry you out.
Remember: it is not just flowers and plants that wilt without
water – humans do too!

REVITALIZE WITH JUICES

Juices extracted from fresh fruit and vegetables are nature's
cure for many ailments. When cooked, fruit and vegetables
lose a lot of their natural goodness as some of the important
vitamins are reduced during the boiling, especially vitamin C
and all the B vitamins which are water-soluble. Processed,
tinned and pre-cooked fruits and vegetables have also lost
much of their natural nutrients.

Naturopathic doctors have used fresh fruit and vegetable
juices for years in their belief that the body can heal itself
through the use of various natural therapies and a healthy diet.
In Switzerland Max Bircher-Benner developed a naturopathic
programme for many diseases and Max Gerson devised the
Gerson therapy in the treatment of cancer. The Rohsafte Kur,
which originated in Germany, is a raw juice fast which is
becoming very popular worldwide as a way of detoxifying the
body and mind and rejuvenating the appearance.

It is important to use fresh vegetables and fruits (organic if
possible) for juicing as most juices sold in bottles, tins or cartons
have in some way been processed or contain preservatives. The
best way of juicing is with an electric juicer. Unfortunately it
does take rather a large quantity of any one fruit or vegetable
to produce just a glass of juice, so it is less expensive to buy
from a market, especially at the end of the day when prices are
dropped for quick sale. However, if buying from a market it is
essential to scrub fruit or vegetables thoroughly as they have
been subjected to pollution and sometimes to many human
hands. Drink homemade juice immediately before the natural
enzymes disperse or pour it into a sealed container and keep
refrigerated for no more than 24 hours. Descriptions follow of
just a few of the many fruits and vegetables you can use for
juicing and you will discover some marvellous cocktails
through mixing them.

BENEFITS OF FRUIT JUICE

Fruit juice is great for so many reasons. It:

• Increases the intake of essential nutrients and trace elements.

• Cleanses the system by its enzymes.

• Can build up red blood cells if it contains chlorophyll, found in leafy green vegetables.

• Counters the effects of stress by strengthening the immune system.

• Defends against infection.

• Improves a sluggish digestive tract.

• Accelerates the assimilation and elimination of accumulated waste.

• Rebalances the body's pH levels.

• Stimulates peristalsis (the rhythmic squeeezing movements through organs such as the intestines if it has a high pectin content, such as that found in apples, oranges and grapefruit.

• Improves skin texture.

• Is easier to digest than whole fruits and vegetables.

• Neutralizes excess proteins and fats by its enzyme content. This also assists the stomach's digestive enzymes to absorb nutrients.

• It has no preservatives, colourings or flavourings.

• May lower cholesterol when pectin-containing fruits are used.

• Increases collagen.

THE FRUITS

APPLE Rich in vitamins C, B1, B2 and B6, beta-carotene, magnesium, sulphur and potassium. Because of its pectin content, apple is beneficial for cleaning out the digestive tract.

GRAPEFRUIT Rich in vitamin C and bioflavonoids (which enhance the action of vitamin C). Also contains calcium, potassium, phosphorus and citric acid.

GRAPES Have a high vitamin C, B1 and B2 content, together with calcium, phosphorus, sulphur and iron. Grapes speed up the metabolism and are therefore useful for weight-loss. They are also very detoxifying.

LEMON Contains more citric acid than any of the other citrus fruits, together with vitamin C. An excellent cleanser, it is also believed to stimulate the liver, which then detoxifies the body. A particular oil found in lemons is thought to help rheumatism. Because of its high acidity, lemon juice should be diluted with water or mixed with other juices as it can wear away tooth enamel.

MANGO A rich source of beta-carotene and vitamin C, together with potassium, magnesium and copper. Fairly high in sugar and should be diluted with water, especially as the juice is very thick.

MELON Orange-fleshed cantaloupe melons are the most nutritious of the melon varieties. They are rich in vitamin C, beta-carotene, vitamins B1, B2 and B6 and folic acid (part of the vitamin B group) together with potassium, phosphorus, magnesium and sulphur. Honeydew melons and watermelons have a lower vitamin and mineral content. All types of melon have a high water content, are cleansers and stimulate the kidneys. Because melon juice is quickly absorbed by the digestive system, it is best drunk on its own.

ORANGE An excellent source of vitamin C and bioflavonoids, together with potassium, zinc, thiamin, folate and phosphorus. Also contains pectin within the pith which is why it is important to juice the fruit with the pith.

PAPAYA (PAW-PAW) Containing a substance called papain, which is a powerful enzyme similar to pepsin, it is important in the breaking down of proteins and fats. It also contains vitamins C, B1, B2 and B3 plus beta-carotene, together with calcium, zinc and potassium.

PEACH Containing vitamin C, folic acid, beta-carotene and calcium, magnesium, potassium and phosphorus, it has a gentle cleansing and laxative effect on the intestines.

PEAR High in natural sugar and a useful source of vitamin C, folic acid, magnesium, calcium and potassium. Also contains a small amount of pectin and is slightly laxative.

PINEAPPLE Contains an enzyme called bromelain which breaks down proteins and can balance acid/alkaline levels within the body. Its main nutrient is vitamin C and it also contains small amounts of folic acid, potassium, sodium and magnesium.

STRAWBERRIES Used in traditional medicine as a way of cleansing and purifying the digestive system, they are also particularly good for cleansing the body tissue and bloodstream. Rich in vitamin C, folic acid and biotin (part of the B group), together with calcium, magnesium, potassium and phosphorus.

• **Citrus fruits are all high in acidity and should be eaten in moderation, especially in cases of urinary tract problems and inflammed joints.**
• **Some people are allergic to citrus fruits and they have been linked to migraine.**
• **Always wash or scrub all fruits and vegetables before using to remove any chemical insecticides.**
• **If you suffer with candidiasis, take fruit only in moderation.**

THE VEGETABLES

BEETROOT Rich in vitamins B1, B2 and B6, folic acid, plus a small amount of vitamin C, and potassium, calcium, magnesium, zinc, phosphorus and sodium. An excellent cleanser, particularly for the liver, gallbladder and kidneys. Its folate content helps to improve red blood cells, useful for anaemia. The red pigment, betacyanin, causes some people's urine to turn pink, but this is no cause for worry. Remove the root.

BROCCOLI Contains vitamin C and beta-carotene, some iron, potassium and folate. The darker the florets, the higher the vitamin C and beta-carotene content. It is a powerful anti-oxidant as well as containing natural fibre.

CARROT Contains vitamins C, D and E and beta-carotene, together with calcium and magnesium. Beneficial for alkalizing the system and rebuilding healthy tissue. It is also a powerful anti-oxidant and mixes well with other juices. Do not peel.

CELERY Especially rich in the minerals potassium, calcium, phosphorus and sodium. Contains an anti-inflammatory substance useful in the treatment of gout. It is a natural diuretic and can help with fluid retention. Use the whole vegetable.

CUCUMBER A mild diuretic containing calcium, potassium, sulphur and folic acid. Its high water content makes it good with other thicker juices. Use the whole vegetable.

SPINACH An excellent source of vitamin C, B6, folic acid and beta-carotene, together with calcium, iron, potassium, sodium, phosphorus and chlorophyll which has anti-bacterial qualities. A marvellous cleansing tonic for the liver and gallbladder, it should not be taken in excess because its oxalic acid content can prevent calcium and iron absorption and could aggravate kidney stone formation in vulnerable cases.

WATERCRESS High in vitamins C, E and beta-carotene, with potassium, magnesium, calcium, phosphorus and sulphur, this is a useful liver and kidney cleanser and a natural antibiotic. It is a member of the crucifer family, together with broccoli, cabbage, Brussels sprouts, kale and cauliflower. Cruciferous plants contain certain phytochemicals which are thought to offer some protection against cancer.

DETOX

If we could look inside our bodies, we would be surprised at the amount of excess wastes and impurities which can accumulate. We are constantly besieged by toxins from internal and external sources.

The body's elimination system, which comprises the liver, kidneys, colon, skin, lungs and lymphatics, works 24 hours a day to filter and cleanse our bodies. However, some toxins can enter the bloodstream and circulate around the tissues and organs, causing a toxic build-up. Poor diet, a sluggish lymphatic system, exposure to pollutants and stress can all exacerbate the situation. As we age our self-cleansing

ONE-DAY CLEANSE

On rising Drink the juice of half a lemon in a glass of warm water.

Breakfast Any fruit from the following: apples, pears, grapes, peaches, mangoes, kiwi fruit and strawberries. It is best to avoid citrus fruits as they will irritate an acid system.

Mid-morning Herb tea (one that does not contain sugar) or freshly squeezed fruit juice diluted with water.

Lunch A vegetable salad made with any of the following: celery, onions, cabbage (red or white), carrots, beetroot, broccoli, lettuce and cauliflower.

Evening meal A mixed vegetable salad followed by a mixed fruit salad from any of the above selections.

Before going to bed Herb tea, preferably camomile or peppermint to relax and soothe the digestive system.

Throughout the day Drink as much water as possible – 1½–2 litres/2½ –3½ pints or more as it will also help to flush out the system.

processes decline and our bodies become overloaded with more toxins than we are able to eliminate. They start to steal from our nutrients, and the result is a congested system. This can cause symptoms, such as fatigue, constipation, skin problems, headaches, recurrent colds and infections.

Detoxifying the body will help to alkalize the system, improve digestion, clear your mind, boost the immune system, improve skin and increase energy. A detox is not a diet, but more a way of inner cleansing – a 'spring-cleaning' of the body.

A detox can last from one day to one month, but if you are detoxing for the first time, it is advisable to start with a one-day plan and repeat it once or twice a month. You may then want to try a two-day plan and repeat it once a month.

Prior to your detox it is best to eat simple foods such as wholegrains, wholewheat pasta and bread, fruits, vegetables, beans and sprouting seeds. This gently prepares the body for its cleanse and should also be repeated after the detox. During the detox you should avoid smoking, coffee, tea, sugar, alcohol, wheat, meat, fish, chocolate and dairy products.

Side effects

Side effects during a detox programme, are a good sign that the toxins are being released. The most common side effect is a headache, and you may also feel colder than usual, lose concentration, feel nauseous and develop smelly breath. Your urine may be darker than usual too. These are all normal symptoms, so do not give up the programme. Avoid taking pain killers or vitamins to enable the liver to rest.

Liver cleansing

The spring, summer and early autumn are good times to work with nature in cleansing the liver. If health problems are associated with liver sluggishness or toxicity, rapid benefit will be felt from a periodic cleansing. Numerous conditions can be caused by or exacerbated by liver sluggishness, such as varicose veins, arthritis, recurring boils, allergies, excessive flatulence and high blood cholesterol levels. The cleansing operation can be carried out over a period varying from one to three weeks and may be repeated periodically if necessary. There are a number of steps to take:

Diet For the period of cleansing follow a largely raw diet incorporating lots of uncooked leafy vegetables, carrots or carrot juice and beetroot, leeks, onions and garlic. Use sprouted grains, especially alfalfa. Add freshly picked dandelion leaves to salads (also good for weeding!) in the spring when they are tender. Dress salads liberally with lemon juice and cold-pressed olive oil. Eat all kinds of fresh fruit, especially grapefruit, but avoid oranges. Moderate consumption of cooked wholegrains and root vegetables is allowable.

Foods to avoid Fried foods, dairy produce, margarines, sugar and foods containing additives should not be eaten. Avoid all meat as it is harder to digest, putting a strain on the liver.

Fluids Do not drink any alcohol, coffee or strong tea. Weak tea with lemon is permissible, and several herbal infusions are beneficial (thyme, rosemary, meadowseet, camomile). Freshly pressed grapefruit juice is helpful for decongesting the liver. Otherwise drink filtered water with fresh lemon juice if desired.

Liver exercise Twice daily place the palm of your hand under the ribcage on the right side of your body and press upwards firmly. Do this ten times, increasing in stages to 20 times.

Olive-oil massage Daily place a little cold-pressed olive oil on the area under the right side of the ribcage and massage gently.

Exercise Regular exercise is valuable as part of a balanced existence and is beneficial during liver cleansing in keeping the blood and lymph circulating freely. Walk, swim or follow your usual exercise routine, trying to raise your pulse rate to about 110–120 beats per minute for about 20 minutes at a time.

What to expect This routine will increase bile elimination and so darkly coloured faeces can be expected, possibly with increased odour. A furred tongue and increased body odour may be noticed, and initially a headache may develop: this suggests that the cleansing is working well, and you will feel much better after the first one or two days when the toxins are eliminated from the body.

TWO-DAY CLEANSE
DAY 1
On rising Drink the juice of half a lemon in a glass of warm water.

For the rest of the day Eat as many grapes (green or black) as possible while drinking plenty of fluids such as the freshly squeezed juices of carrot and celery or apple and papaya. Do not mix the fruit and vegetable juices and always dilute the fruit juice with water. Include the 1½–2 litres/2½–3½ pints of water throughout the day as for the one-day cleanse and always rinse the mouth after eating grapes otherwise they can affect tooth enamel.

DAY 2
On rising Drink the juice of half a lemon in a glass of warm/hot water.

For the rest of the day Eat as many apples or pears as possible. Keep drinking the diluted fruit and vegetable juices and water, and to these add herb tea, finishing with a relaxing camomile tea before bed.

Additional ways of detoxifying

Body brushing Body brushing stimulates the lymphatic system and clears the skin of dead cells. It is important to use a pure bristle brush, not a nylon one. Always beginning at the feet, use upward-sweeping movements in the direction of the heart. Brush all over the body apart from the face. In the neck area brush downwards towards the heart. Be careful around the breast and do not brush broken or irritated skin. Body brushing is good before a bath or shower and can be repeated about three times a week.

Epsom salt baths Made from magnesium sulphate. Epsom salts draw impurities from the skin. Add 225g/8oz of Epsom salts to a hot bath and soak for 20 minutes. Be sure to wrap up well after the bath as your body will continue to perspire and eliminate toxins for several hours. Drink lots of water during this time. Epsom salt baths should not be used if you suffer with eczema. Try an oatmeal bath instead. Fill a muslin bag with porridge oats and hang over the hot tap while the water is running. Then float the bag in the bath while you soak for about 20 minutes. Allow your skin to dry naturally.

Massage Treat yourself to a lymphatic drainage or aromatherapy massage or use a few drops of juniper, cypress and lemon essential oils to your morning bath or rose and camomile to your evening bath. These combinations are both detoxifying and aid digestion.

FOOD ALLERGY & INTOLERANCE

An allergy is any reaction to a food or substance in the environment which gives rise to an immune response. A food intolerance is a reaction to a particular food and although the immune system may be involved, it is not a major factor.

Food allergy

For a food to be described as an allergen (an allergy-causing substance which the body regards as alien and therefore harmful) 30 or 40 years ago, there had to be an instantaneous response to it, often swelling of the lips and mouth, nausea

CAUSES

Common causes of food allergy are:

• Milk.

• Wheat.

• Gluten.

• Shellfish.

• Eggs.

• Nuts (especially peanuts).

• Sugar.

• Food additives.

and, in the more severe cases, anaphylactic shock (due mainly to a sudden release of histamine into the system causing a rapid drop in blood pressure, swelling of the mucus membranes of the throat and spasm in the bronchi). There had to be a positive prick test for a definite diagnosis to be made.

In the 1960s immunoglobin E (IgE) was discovered, and proved to be the main culprit in allergy. The measurement of the level of this antibody to a specific allergen was carried out through the Rast (radioallergosorbent) test, developed during this time. It enabled true food allergies to be pinpointed. The main purpose of IgE is to protect the body from parasitic invasion. The IgE molecules attach themselves to mast cells (connective tissue cells which do not circulate in the blood), which are more commonly found around the nasal passages, bronchi and intestines – areas often vulnerable to allergy.

Dr James Braly of the Research Institute in Florida, Immuno Laboratories, has developed a new test based on a different antibody called IgG. He believes delayed food allergies are the inability of the digestive tract to prevent large quantities of undigested food from entering the bloodstream. As understanding of our immune system and technology develop, conventional theory will be constantly disputed.

Although most allergies begin at an early age, the initial exposure to any particular allergen cannot cause a reaction because no antibodies have yet been formed. Food allergies can be responsible for any of the classic allergy diseases, such as asthma, eczema, hayfever, rhinitis, urticaria (nettle rash), skin irritation, runny or itchy eyes, sneezing or wheezing.

People can be allergic to foods that are rarely eaten and, unlike in cases of food intolerance, they do not crave the offending food. Even the tiniest particle of an offending food can cause an allergic reaction.

Food allergies can affect the mind as well as the body. Dr Abraham Hoffer, a Canadian researcher and formerly Professor of Psychiatry at the University of Saskatchewan, has been researching the effects of diet on mental health since the 1950s. Having treated around 5,000 mentally ill patients, he

PHYSICAL SYMPTOMS OF FOOD ALLERGY OR INTOLERANCE

- Eczema or skin rashes.
- Asthma or hayfever.
- Blocked nose, rhinitis, catarrh and sinus problems.
- Ear infections and tonsillitis, especially in children.
- Swollen hands, face and eyes.
- Bloating and IBS.
- Headaches and migraines.
- Painful swelling of the joints.
- Weight gain.
- Increased appetite.
- Coeliac disease (insensitivity to gluten).

MENTAL SYMPTOMS OF FOOD ALLERGY OR INTOLERANCE

- Depression and anxiety.
- Mood swings.
- Lack of concentration.
- Dyslexia or learning difficulties in children.
- Hyperactivity in children.
- Tiredness and lethargy, especially after meals.

estimates that half of them have food allergies, the common offenders being dairy products, wheat, sugar, tea and coffee.

Homeopathy can often help with allergy problems, but be prepared to make changes to your diet. Certain Bach Flower Remedies may be useful (see page 108).

Food intolerance

Food intolerance differs from food allergy in many ways. With intolerance the reaction can be many hours or even days later. The reaction will be to foods that are eaten regularly, and larger amounts are needed to provoke intolerance. The offending food is often craved, but it can eventually become tolerated if it is avoided for a long time. With intolerance the symptoms vary and may come and go.

Complete digestion is an important contribution to preventing food intolerance. Any deficiency of digestive enzymes or specific chemical products needed for complete digestion will cause problems. For example, if proteins are not broken down correctly into simple amino acids, these incompletely digested particles become toxic to the cells. If the body's ability to eliminate these toxins is functioning properly then there is no problem; if it is not, food sensitivity is often the result. Other factors which lend a hand to food intolerance are PMT, hormonal imbalance, hypoglycaemia (low blood sugar) and stress. An elimination diet is usually the best way of identifying the culprit food.

COMMON SYMPTOMS OF MILK & DAIRY INTOLERANCE

• Abdominable bloating, including constipation, diarrhoea, migraine (especially from cheese) and eczema.

• Milk is mucus-forming, which sometimes causes chest problems such as catarrh and wheezing.

• Babies with this intolerance may be prone to colic, wind and catarrh.

COMMON OFFENDING FOODS

Milk and dairy produce Butter, cream, cheese, yoghurt, ice cream cause food allergy or intolerance in some people. Milk is one of the most common culprits as it contains lactose (milk sugar) which many people are unable to digest satisfactorily. As babies we have enough lactase (an enzyme present in the cells of the small intestine), to assist the digestion of lactose, but as we grow older the natural supply becomes diminished and this can result in an intolerance, causing various health problems.

Beware also of lactose- and whey-containing foods. Milk is a high source of calcium, so it is important to include other calcium-rich foods in the diet when excluding milk. Substitute with calcium-enriched soya milk, goat or sheep's milk, soya-based cheese, soya desserts, creams, yoghurts and ghee (clarified butter made from vegetable oils).

Wheat and gluten Unfortunately wheat is a very common cause of allergy symptoms as it forms a large percentage of the average diet. It can provide vitamin C, most of the B vitamins, iron and fibre, but it can also bring on many problems. One of the main culprits with wheat intolerance is its gluten content. This sticky substance is particularly hard to digest, which can then increase the growth of candida albicans, causing toxicity in the bowel. Gluten is also found in rye, oats and barley. Some people are allergic to gluten and not wheat alone or perhaps both.

Checking labels is important when you are trying to exclude wheat from your diet. Some suggested substitutes for wheat are buckwheat, rye, oats and oatcakes (these contain gluten), wheat-free pasta such as egg pasta, rice cakes. Gluten free breads, cakes and cereals are available nowadays.

Yeast Yeast is found in all alcohol, stock cubes, marmite, vinegar and of course bread. Sufferers from candidiasis are particularly prone to yeast intolerance and should be aware of their consumption of cheese, mushrooms, malt and peanuts, which are part of the same family. An alternative to bread is soda bread or sourdough bread. There are yeast-free products available in some health-food shops.

Eggs Allergy to eggs has a lot to do with the type of feed the hens were given, which sometimes includes maize, wheat and special dyes to make the yolks more yellow. Ascertain whether the allergy is to the chicken feed or to the eggs themselves which then means you could be allergic to chicken also. Look for egg-free products.

COMMON SYMPTOMS OF WHEAT & GLUTEN INTOLERANCE
- Digestive problems.
- IBS.
- Arthritis.
- Tiredness and lethargy.
- Headaches and migraine.
- Coelic disease (an intolerance specifically to gluten).
- Depression.

COMMON SYMPTOMS OF YEAST INTOLERANCE
- Thrush.
- Cystitis.
- Digestive problems.
- Sugar and alcohol cravings.
- Depression and lethargy.

COMMON SYMPTOMS OF EGG INTOLERANCE
- Stomach upset.
- Skin rash.
- Eczema.
- Asthma.

COMMON SYMPTOMS OF
EXCESS CAFFEINE INTAKE

- Upset stomach.
- Headaches.
- Migraines.
- Insomnia.
- Palpitations.
- Rapid breathing.
- Sweating.
- Hyperactivity in children.

CAUTION

Caffeine should be avoided or intake
greatly reduced in cases of:

- High blood pressure.
- Heart problems.
- Kidney disease.
- Pregnancy and lactation (foetuses
can absorb caffeine).
- Osteoporosis (caffeine increases
calcium excretion).
- Gastric ulcers.
- Digestive problems.
- Hiatus hernia (caffeine stimulates
the secretion of stomach acid).

OTHER MAJOR OFFENDERS

Caffeine Discovered back in 1827, having been chemically
isolated in 1820, caffeine is a natural constituent of more than
60 plants. Coffee and tea are the obvious sources, but it is also
found in certain colas and other soft drinks, chocolate, cocoa,
many 'instant energy' drinks, guarana, some cold and pain relief
remedies and certain diuretics.

Once it has been consumed, caffeine is rapidly absorbed into
the bloodstream and into all the body fluids, including saliva,
semen, breast milk and bile. It is then transported to all the
major body organs, reaching its peak of effectiveness about an
hour after ingestion. In the brain, caffeine affects the
neurotransmitters (chemical messengers) and stimulates the
central nervous system. This increases awareness by triggering
the release of adrenaline into the bloodstream and raising
blood sugar levels. Caffeine also stimulates the kidneys.

This quick 'fix' raises alertness, improves concentration and
generally increases mental and physical performance –
temporarily. After an hour or two the blood sugar levels start to
drop, eventually plummeting to a lower point than before.
Feeling the need for another 'lift', many people then tend to
have another cup of coffee or reach for biscuits, chocolate or
any food which will raise the blood sugar and energy
superficially. The caffeine content in tea can have a similar
effect although to a lesser degree. Theophylline, another
stimulant found in coffee and tea is often responsible for
problems associated with caffeine.

Decaffeinated versions of these drinks are now widely
available, but even after decaffeinating there usually remains
about 2–3 per cent caffeine in the products, so if you are trying
to cut down they will ease withdrawal symptoms such as
headaches, lethargy, poor concentration and irritability.
Dandelion coffee is another useful alternative.

As well as caffeine, tea contains tannic acid, which can also
irritate the digestive system. Additionally it has been
suggested that tea can decrease the absorption of iron from
foods. Luaka tea has the lowest tannin and caffeine content.

Salt Originally salt was used as a preservative, but over the years we have grown used to it as a flavour enhancer. It still preserves food, yet at the same time it makes it harder to digest.

The type of salt used in cooking or at the dinner table is sodium chloride. Sodium on the other hand is a mineral occurring naturally in all foods which our bodies need – in minimal amounts. We need sodium for our cells to function properly, to maintain healthy blood pressure, to regulate fluid balance together with potassium, and for correct muscular and neurological functioning. Without sodium we would die.

We should obtain all the sodium we need from foods such as vegetables, fruit, cereals and milk and there should be no need for extra salt to be added during cooking or at the table. We can avoid adding salt to food we prepare ourselves, but large amounts are 'hidden' in many pre-prepared foods: preservatives, additives for emulsifying, flavouring and stabilizers. Surprisingly a bowl of cornflakes, for example, is usually packed full of salt and contains 444mg of sodium compared to a 35g/1½oz packet of crisps which contains 375mg. All tinned, pre-cooked and packet foods contain salt unless stated otherwise. Sodium can also be found in chocolate, treacle, golden syrup, toffee, tomato juice, soda water, mineral water and some bedtime malted drinks.

People who exercise a lot, such as athletes, dancers and sportspeople, will probably need more sodium as they lose it through perspiration.

There are many ways of giving flavour to food other than with salt. Using herbs (see page 211) is far healthier. Low-sodium salt is available from most health-food shops and supermarkets, but should be avoided by diabetics or anyone prone to kidney problems as it contains potassium which should be kept at a low level in both conditions.

Sea-salt is produced by evaporating sea water and it contains small amounts of minerals, including iodine, so is a healthier option than ordinary sodium chloride. Bio Salt, a biochemically balanced mineral salt compound is also available; this, however, does not contain lactose.

COMMON SYMPTOMS OF EXCESS SODIUM INTAKE

• High blood pressure which can lead to heart and kidney disease.

• Pre-menstrual bloating and fluid retention.

• Adrenal exhaustion

• Risk of developing osteoporosis due to the increase in calcium excretion.

COMMON SYMPTOMS OF EXCESS SUGAR INTAKE

- Diabetes.
- Hypoglycaemia.
- Arthritis.
- Cancer.
- Heart disease.
- Tooth decay and periodontal disease.
- Allergies.
- Asthma.
- Osteoporosis.
- Headaches.
- Digestive problems.
- Candidiasis.
- Immunity to infection.
- Hyperactivity (especially in children).

Sugar Sugar is sweetness without substance; it is nutritionally worthless and full of 'empty' calories.

At the turn of the century the average person in the USA ate 4.5–9kg/10–20lb of sugar per year according to Dr Ray Wunderlich Jr MD. By 1982, when he published *Sugar and Your Health*, the amount had risen to as much as 54.5kg/120lb per person per year. Sugar consumption figures continue to rise both in the USA and Europe.

There are various kinds of sugar. The most obvious to us all, table sugar or sucrose, is the main ingredient of sugar cane and sugar beet. Other kinds of sugar are fructose, found in fruit and honey; lactose from milk; multose in sprouting grains; and glucose, also found in fruit, honey and vegetables. The sweetest form is fructose.

Sugar is one of the main types of carbohydrate (the other is starch) which provide us with energy. Sugar is broken down into glucose during digestion and released into the bloodstream, providing fuel for the muscles, cells and organs. It is important that the correct levels of glucose are maintained in the blood. The pancreas is responsible for this by secreting insulin, which transports glucose from the blood into the cells. If the body is unable to regulate its blood sugar levels, as in the case of diabetes, hypoglycaemia (low blood sugar) or hyperglycaemia (high blood sugar) can result.

Sucrose and glucose are absorbed straight into the bloodstream, raising the level of blood sugar very quickly. We get an immediate 'sugar rush' from this, but then the blood sugar level falls just as quickly after a short while, which then makes us feel lethargic. A similar cycle to the caffeine cycle then begins, during which we need more sugar to lift us out of the 'sugar blues' and so the whole pattern starts over again.

According to Nancy Appleton in her book *Lick the Sugar Habit*: Every time we ingest two teaspoons of sugar the mineral ratios in our bodies change. The vitamins and minerals in our bodies are always changing – that is what homeostasis (maintenance of our internal equilibrium) involves, a continual fine tuning of the body chemistry. Sugar causes these micronutrients to change radically, throwing the blood chemistry out of homeostasis. When minerals are out of balance day after day, year after year the ability of the body to balance back into homeostasis is exhausted. The body can no longer fine tune itself.

Excess sugar in the diet can have a number of bad effects. It strips calcium from the bones and teeth and is then deposited into the joints, muscles, arteries and organs. This can lead to a whole host of problems. The thyroid and adrenal functions are also reduced by sugar. Viruses, yeasts, bacteria and fungi all love a sweet digestive system.

Although brown sugar and honey may have a healthier image than white sugar, they are still concentrated sugars and should be consumed in extreme moderation. Honey contains glucose, fructose and a little sucrose along with a small quantity of vitamins, minerals and enzymes. It is generally absorbed more slowly than sugar. Brown sugar is often white sugar with a little molasses added to give it colour. Blackstrap molasses is a healthy alternative to sugar as it is rich in calcium, phosphorus, chromium and zinc.

Eating plenty of complex carbohydrates such as potatoes, wholegrain breads, pasta, vegetables, rice and oats, will help to control blood sugar levels. Eating little and often is also beneficial, in preventing dramatic fluctuations in blood sugar. Watch out for all those 'hidden' sugars in tinned fruits, cereals, sauces and alcohol.

Artificial sweeteners Artificial sweeteners are found in many diet drinks and desserts as well as in table-top sweeteners. They include saccharin, aspartame, sorbitol, mannitol, xylitol, cyclamate and acesulfame K. Most of them are 200–400 times sweeter than sugar.

Saccharin and aspartame are the two most commonly used. Aspartame, discovered in 1965, is 200 times sweeter than sugar. The British government has passed it as non-toxic, but seven other European countries continue to prohibit its use. Regarding, saccharin, also considered to be safe by the government, questions were raised concerning cancer when it was tested on animals.

The use of these sweeteners has rocketed in Britain, By 1993 we used 801,000 tonnes of aspartame and 1,000,000 tonnes of saccharin. The Food Commission found these sweeteners in children's lollies and jellies, crisps, puddings and tinned pasta and are now calling for a reduction in their use and clear labelling on all products containing artificial sweeteners.

BALANCING YOUR SUGAR

There are a number of ways in which you can help your blood sugar balance to keep steady:

• Cut down on refined carbohydrates and stimulants.

• Avoid sugar and sugary foods.

• Eat little and often and never miss breakfast.

• Dilute fruit juice with water.

• Avoid alcohol, tea and coffee (even decaffeinated coffee).

• Avoid honey – remember that it is also a refined sugar.

• Include adequate protein in the diet.

• Avoid becoming overweight.

• Take regular physical exercise.

The glucose tolerance factor A body constantly overfed with sugar develops a 'trigger-happy' pancreas and the result is a feeling of lethargy known as hypoglycaemia (low blood sugar). To deal with excessive sugar intake the pancreas first reacts by producing too much insulin, which causes the blood sugar to drop rapidly. If the pancreas is overstimulated too often, however, it becomes exhausted and consequently produces too little insulin resulting in hyperglycaemia (high blood sugar). In its most acute form this becomes diabetes.

To keep the insulin 'scales' balanced the aim is to provide all the cells, including the brain, with enough energy, while at the same time preventing unwanted glucose from remaining in the blood. If the balance is inclined even slightly, both physical and mental health can suffer. The symptoms can include depression, dizziness or light-headedness, headaches, insomnia, digestive problems, allergies, lack of libido, lethargy, lack of concentration and irritability.

WAYS OF TESTING FOOD SENSITIVITY

Exclusion diet An exclusion diet is one of the most reliable ways of discovering food intolerances. It simply excludes one or more suspect foods for a period of time and then gradually reintroduces the foods into the diet.

It is best to follow this diet for a period of ten days to three weeks depending on the time the food takes to leave the system. If symptoms improve or disappear, it means the excluded food was contributing to your problems, if there is no change, it means that the excluded food was not the cause.

The next stage, if symptoms have improved, is to reintroduce the particular food or food group into your diet, usually after about 14 days. Reintroduction should be at intervals of about three to seven days. Carefully monitor your own symptoms: a reaction to a food can occur within minutes, but generally happens after several hours or even days. If there is a reaction, continue to exclude that food for at least a month. With luck the symptoms will improve again until the next reintroduction, when you will be able to assess whether the first reaction was real or superficial. Once you have pinpointed the culprit food avoid it for several months and then try it again. Initially you may feel worse when excluding certain foods due to withdrawal, but symptoms will soon disappear.

The exclusion diet can be a long process and ideally should be carried out under the expert guidance of a nutritionist as a vitamin or mineral deficiency may arise because of the exclusion of certain food(s). However, if you are suffering from any of the food intolerance symptoms, your commitment will be rewarded by a discovery which will improve your health, increase your energy and allow your body time to heal itself.

Vega testing Vega testing uses electrical probes, which are usually attached to the fingers or toes, as a way of measuring the body's electromagnetic reaction to certain foods.

Systematic kinesiology Using a system of muscle testing a qualified kinesiologist can detect allergenic foods as they cause certain muscles to weaken. Kinesiology can also detect any imbalance within the body such as hormonal or digestive.

Rast test The rast test (radiallergosorbent) picks up only true food allergies in which the immune system is involved, and not intolerances. It identifies specific blood antibodies to problem foods and substances such as pollen, dust and moulds.

Skin prick test This test also detects IgE reactions but is more beneficial for skin allergies than food allergies.

MINOR OFFENDERS

As well as the major offenders listed on page 200 onwards, an exclusion diet often pinpoints an intolerance to:
• Shellfish which can bring on stomach upsets and migraine.
• Soya which can sometimes cause indigestion and headaches.
• Nuts which can cause asthma, eczema, rashes and, in severe cases, anaphylactic shock.
• Food additives tartrazine, a colouring agent, and the preservative benzoic acid, are among the many food additives found in processed and take-away foods and have been attributed to hyperactivity and certain changes in behaviour.

Cytotoxic Test Cytotoxic means 'toxic to the cells' and this test is designed to measure changes in the activity of the neutrophils, through taking a sample of blood.

ELISA Test ELISA stands for 'Enzyme Linked Immuno Sorbent Assay'. It was developed by Dr. James Braly in the Immuno Laboratories (see page 197) as a way of testing IgG reactions to allergens. It is a proven method for detecting HIV positivity.

Allergy of any sort usually signifies an imbalance in a person's lifestyle, and those listed are just some of the methods used for testing. None of these techniques is 100 per cent accurate and more tests are continually being researched.

HELPFUL NUTRITIONAL ACCESSORIES

Pro-biotics Pro-biotics literally meaning pro-life, are supplements which contain friendly bacteria necessary for a healthy colon. Under normal circumstances the colon contains a large amount of friendly bacteria, or 'flora', which assist the process of digestion and controls infection from the harmful bacteria, yeasts and moulds.

When we take a course of antibiotics for bacterial infection of some kind (perhaps a severe throat infection), unfortunately the friendly bacteria are also destroyed in the process, which then paves the way for the undesirable bacteria, yeasts and moulds to repopulate. The result can be numerous digestive disorders such as constipation, IBS and diarrhoea, as well as skin disorders, muscular problems, headaches, migraines, arthritis and candidiasis. Supplementing the diet with pro-biotics which contain beneficial bacteria, such as lactobacilli and bifidobacteria, can often help with these conditions and is indeed advisable after a course of antibiotics. Acidophilus bifidus is now an ingredient in some brands of yoghurt.

Cider vinegar Made from fermented apple juice, cider vinegar has been used for years and is believed to have numerous therapeutic properties. Many naturopaths believe that it can help alleviate the symptoms of arthritis, gout, rheumatism, hayfever, asthma, digestive problems, high blood pressure, coughs, sore throats and insomnia. It is also believed to improve the condition of the skin, hair, nails and eyes. Additionally it normalizes metabolism which can sometimes benefit slimmers.

The recommended dosage is one or two teaspoons of cider vinegar in a glass of warm water either first thing in the morning on an empty stomach, or twice a day with meals. Many people find that the addition of a teaspoon of clear unblended honey makes ths sour taste a little more palatable. Cider vinegar should be avoided by those with a yeast sensitivity and by regular sufferers of indigestion.

Garlic This little miracle bulb is known to have been used as far back as 1500 BC by the Egyptians to treat many forms of physical weakness. In the Second World War British physicians used garlic to treat battle wounds. It contains sulphur compounds, one of which, allicin, is responsible for its pungent odour. It is these compounds which are responsible for its numerous medicinal properties. It is anti-bacterial, anti-fungal and antiviral and is beneficial for fighting infection, controlling fat and cholesterol levels, improving the health of the digestive system and destroying harmful bacteria and fungi such as candida. It has also been known to help lower blood pressure and maintain a healthy heart.

It is best eaten raw, but is also a tasty addition to food. If you find it totally unpalatable, try garlic capsules.

Aloe vera Aloe vera is one variety of the aloe, of which there are around 300 different varieties in total. This cactus-like plant has been used medicinally for thousands of years, initially by the Greeks, Romans, Chinese and Egyptians, and during biblical times. Today it is grown mainly in Mexico, Texas and the Philippines.

Aloe gel, derived from the leaf of the plant, is a common ingredient in skin creams because of its moisturizing benefits.

The gel is also extremely beneficial for healing wounds and soothing skin burns.

Aloe juice, made from different parts of the plant, can be taken internally and is said to have numerous benefits. It has been effective in cases of arthritis, IBS, eczema, psoriasis, herpes, food sensitivities, candidiasis, stomach ulcers, gingivitis, constipation and ME. It also has detoxifying, anti-inflammatory and immune-stimulating properties, which make the aloe vera little short of a miracle plant.

The secret of the miraculous powers of aloe vera lies in its high content of mucopolysaccharides, vital substances found in our body cells which we are able to manufacture until our teenage years, but after which we have to obtain from plant sources. These mucopolysaccharides are important for lubricating the joints and lining the large intestinal wall, protecting it against toxic waste. Aloe also contains vitamins B1, B2, B3, and B6, vitamins C and E, iron, magnesium, calcium, zinc, numerous fatty acids and amino acids.

The leaf of the fresh plant is highly effective when applied on the skin, otherwise prepared skin-care products are available from some health-food shops together with the juice. It is better to purchase the real juice rather than the watered-down extract.

Pregnant women should not take aloe and diabetics should be carefully monitored if they with to try it.

Royal jelly Royal jelly is a white jelly-like substance produced by the very young worker bees to feed the selected larvae that eventually become queens. It is an excellent supplement and is the richest natural source of pantothenic acid in particular. It also contains all the other B vitamins, amino acids, minerals and enzymes. Research in Bulgaria has found it to be beneficial for lowering high blood pressure and cholesterol, stimulating the immune system, combatting depression, skin problems, insomnia and hayfever and repairing damaged tissue. The fresh royal jelly is the most active but unfortunately is harder to find. It is more readily available in capsules, though has, of course, undergone processing to reach this form.

Propolis Propolis is a resinous substance made from leaves and tree bark by honey bees to bind together their hives. It is rich in bioflavonoids which are anti-viral substances and it also has some anti-inflammatory properties. It may benefit the immune system against colds, flu and periodontal disease. Scientists are still researching its effectiveness in preventing cancer. Propolis can be obtained from most health-food shops either in honey, capsules or lozenges (especially good for sore throats).

Pollen Gathered by the bees in the process of collecting nectar for honey, pollen is one of nature's most perfect foods and contains a rich supply of water-soluble vitamins including B12 and C. It also contains beta-carotene, vitamins E and K, 19 amino acids, various minerals and rutin which is important for collagen formation. Pollen is very beneficial for skin problems and general dryness, and may also help hayfever and minor infections. It is available from most health-food shops in tablet or capsule form.

Evening primrose oil Evening primrose oil is one of the richest sources of gamma linoleic acid, which is needed for the production of prostoglandins (active hormone substances in the body). It can reduce inflammation and lower cholesterol and high blood pressure. It can give relief from joint pain, such as that experienced with arthritis, and is extremely beneficial for skin conditions such as eczema. Menopausal symptoms such as hot flushes and vaginal dryness and menstrual symptoms such as heavy bleeding, cramps and backache may be alleviated by its use.

Co-enzyme Q10 Co-enzyme Q10 (Ubiquinone), a very good anti-oxidant, is found in every cell in the body. It is essential for promoting the course of action for energy production in the mitochondria of the cells. Levels of co-enzyme Q10 decrease as we age, although physical fitness can help to raise them. The Japanese have been taking co-enzyme Q10 for many years and are researching its benefits in treating heart conditions and high blood pressure. Deficiency states may occur in the elderly, possibly due to poor diet and stress; and they are linked to heart disease and loss of energy. Because of its anti-oxidant effects co-enzyme Q10 may be of value in slowing the ageing process and increasing immune strength. It has also been shown to be effective treatment for gingivitis.

Chlorella With its high chlorophyll, zinc and iron content and 19 of the 22 amino acids, chlorella is one of nature's most active natural cleansers and detoxifiers. It is also particularly rich in RNA and DNA, important to growth, metabolism, reproduction and protein synthesis. Its high vitamin B12 content makes it beneficial for vegetarians.

Kelp Kelp, a type of seaweed, is a wonderful source of iodine and is often recommended for thyroid-related problems. It also contains vitamin K, which is currently being researched for its role in the prevention for osteoporosis.

Green superfoods Green superfoods, some of nature's most nutritious foods, have a high content of vitamins and minerals, trace minerals, enzymes and some amino acids. They have remarkable cleansing and balancing effects on the system because of their alkalinity.

Spirulina Containing 60 per cent usable protein with all the essential amino acids, this blue-green alga is also a very rich source of beta-carotene, iron, calcium, vitamin B12 and chlorophyll. It is the only food besides mother's milk which contains the essential fatty acid GLA.

Spirulina is easy to digest and absorb and has a beneficial effect on the immune system. Shipments of this wonder food were sent to Chernobyl after the accident at the nuclear power, station since when Soviet doctors have reported an improvement in the health of the local children due to a boost to their T cells. Now it is being tested by NASA for use in long-term space missions.

Barley and wheatgrass These young cereal grasses barley and wheatgrass contain vitamin C, a rich profile of B vitamins and around 25 per cent protein with eight essential amino acids. They are low in fat and calories and contain no wheat gluten. The powders from these grasses provide more dietary fibre than bran for good colon health and regularity and are especially useful for people who do not eat enough leafy green vegetables.

Glucosamine Glucosamine, an amino sugar which is manufactured in the body, is one of the primary constituents of synovial fluid. However, glucosamine has far wider potentials than muscles and joints. It is advisable to take this substance in the form of glucosamine sulfate as it is non-toxic and it is the sulphur which is the essential part of the molecule during tissue remodelling. The most recent form of glucosamine to become available is called chrondroitin, and for optimal prevention of damage to joints and eyes it is recommended that it be taken in conjunction with a diet high in anti-oxidant supplementation to prevent free radical reactions.

Although still relatively unheard of, glucosamine could prove to be a winner for the future.

THE HEALING POWER OF HERBS

Herbs existed long before humans appeared on the planet, and today herbal medicine can be viewed as the forerunner of pharmacology. Herbalism dates back several thousand years when just a few hundred herbs were used for healing in countries such as China, India and Greece. Today the number of plants with known medicinal properties has expanded into the thousands, and the knowledge associated with these plants has been passed from generation to generation.

Most of Britain's knowledge of herbs stems from that of the ancient Egyptians. The Romans were also practitioners of herbal medicine, and in fact it was the Roman conquerors of Europe who brought lavender and rosemary to Britain, among many other Mediterranean herbs. In India herbal medicine plays a large part in ayurvedic medicine which is based on the belief that the

Herbal preparations are widely available in health-food shops and chemists nowadays but there are some cautions to be considered:
• If you are taking long-term medication prescribed by your doctor, tell your herbalist before you receive treatment from him.
• If you are suffering with any acute condition such as digestive upsets, coughs or headaches and symptoms do not improve or become worse after a few days, it is best to seek professional help.
• During pregnancy, avoid the following: agnus castus, angelica, astragalus, bearberry, coltsfoot, sage, cowslip, devil's claw, fennel, feverfew, ginseng and peppermint.
• During pregnancy the following should only be taken externally: arnica, comfrey, red clove.
• The following herbs should not be given to children: agnus castus, angelica, astragalus, bearberry, devil's claw, sage, feverfew, ginseng and peppermint. Arnica and comfrey should be used only externally.

use of herbs together with a controlled diet can restore homeostasis. The Chinese have various schools of herbal medicine and it is used widely in hospitals today. They believe that illness results from physical or mental conflict and that, together with acupuncture, Chinese herbs can enable the body to heal itself. Chinese herbs have become extremely popular in the west and many qualified practitioners are using them.

In fact modern orthodox doctors rely very much on plant-based medication and, although the therapeutic effects of herbs have not been proved scientifically, continuing research may identify new active plant ingredients which will create the foundation for drugs to combat cancer and Aids. The active substance is in a living relationship with other plant ingredients.

Aspirin is probably the best-known orthdox medication which is plant-based. The word aspirin is derived from the Latin *a spireae,* meaning 'out of meadowsweet'. Meadowsweet contains salicylates similar in composition to aspirin and can be used symptomatically in much the same way as aspirin (as can willow bark). In the 1830s salicin was first extracted from willow bark. Aspirin was eventually produced in a laboratory in 1857.

One of the most renowned British herbalists was Nicholas Culpeper (1616–54), who wrote several books on the subject, and today there still exist some shops named after him selling herbal preparations. In 1812 Henry Potter began to supply herbs in London. By this time different herbs were being used in combination with one another and not just individually. Henry Potter's family business still exists today.

Who can benefit from herbs?

Anyone can benefit from the use of herbs, although the dosage will vary in children and the elderly. Many herbs are safe to take during pregnancy except where indicated; however, it is wise to take them only when they are really needed. Herbal medicines can help all kinds of conditions, including arthritis, skin problems, digestive disorders, respiratory conditions, headaches, migraines, high blood pressure, urinary tract conditions, menopause, insomnia, stress, menstrual problems and ME.

MEDICINAL HERBS

The best way of using herbs is in your daily diet, but if you are taking a particular herb for a specific condition, the small amount from an average daily diet may not contain enough of the nutritional value. It is then beneficial to take herbal supplements. This is a selection of commonly used herbs together with their benefits.

AGNUS CASTUS Works on the pituitary gland to balance the secretions of oestrogens and progesterones. It is helpful for PMT, bloating, breast tenderness and mood swings. Used in conjunction with St John's wort, it is very beneficial for menopause, although there is very little point in taking agnus castus if you are on HRT. It can also be useful following hysterectomy.

ANGELICA Warming, improves circulation to the hands, feet and digestive organs. Good also for anaemia. Chinese angelica (dong quai) is a very important herb for women's health. It balances oestrogen levels and is therefore beneficial for menstrual and menopausal problems. It can be taken in association with HRT to soothe osteoporosis. It has vascular benefits, is a powerful muscle relaxant and has been known to relax muscular contractions.

ARNICA Good for muscle aches, bruises, joint pain and sprains.

ASTRAGALUS A Chinese herb which has powerful effects on the immune system: it can increase white blood cell production. It is an adaptogen which can help the body to adapt to stress. It is anti-bacterial and can reduce the duration of a cold. It has been used successfully in the treatment of ME.

BEARBERRY A urinary antiseptic, good for cystitis, but not for kidney problems.

BURDOCK Beneficial for removing toxicity, chronic skin problems. The root used in conjunction with dandelion root is beneficial for acne and boils. Burdock is also a mild diuretic.

CAMOMILE Known as the 'mother of the gut', it is anti-inflammatory and beneficial for IBS and stress-induced digestive problems. It is very relaxing and therefore beneficial for insomnia, although some people may need to try limeflowers or even valerian if camomile fails to work for them. It is safe for children.

CLEAVERS Diuretic, decongests the lymphatic system, good for chronic skin conditions.

COLTSFOOT Good for respiratory problems such as bronchitis, catarrh and asthma.

COMFREY Also known as knitbone, which literally describes its action – it has been used to heal fractures. It is anti-inflammatory, containing allantoin which attracts white blood cells to areas which are damaged. It has been used for osteoarthritis and the ointment is particularly beneficial for arthritic joints, although it should not be used for liver problems. Comfrey diluted in water makes a wonderful liquid manure for gardeners.

CORNSILK Beneficial for cystitis and water retention.

COWSLIP The flower is a useful sedative and the leaves have expectorant properties which can help bronchitis. Cowslip is also beneficial for rheumatic problems.

CRAMP BARK A good anti-spasmodic, this can be used for muscle tension, colic, muscle cramps and restless legs.

DANDELION A good liver tonic and can be beneficial for hangovers. It is also very diuretic and can help constipation, acne and allergies. Dandelion is suitable for children. Whereas orthodox diuretics can have side effects, dandelion is readily absorbed. It contains huge amounts of potassium which helps to maintain normal fluid levels in the body. It is therefore beneficial for ankle oedema and general fluid retention. Roasted dandelion root can be ground and made into coffee.

DEVIL'S CLAW Anti-inflammatory, if taken with celery seeds it stimulates the kidneys to detoxify. Devil's claw is beneficial for osteoarthritis and rheumatoid arthritis.

ECHINACEA A wonder herb with powerful effects on the immune system, this was originally used in North America for treating snake bites. It inhibits the spread of viruses as it contains hyaluronidase, a substance actually found in snake bite. It increases the production of white blood cells, which is why it is such a powerful immune stimulant. It can also speed the healing of wounds. Proved beneficial for throat infections, tonsillitis, acne, boils, candidiasis, glandular fever, flu and ME, it can be taken with antibiotics to reduce their side effects.

ELDERFLOWER Good for colds, coughs, hayfever, bronchitis, catarrh, sinus problems, sore throats, eye problems and, for children, teething, infections and nosebleeds. As an eyebath use elderflower tea lukewarm. Babies should use a quarter of the adult dose and children half. Adults should drink six cups of elderflower tea daily for two to four days.

EYEBRIGHT Anti-catarrhal, it can be beneficial for colds, flu, earache and eye problems. Mixed with elderflower, it can give the best results for conditions such as hayfever and catarrh. It is good for any chronic mucus problems.

FENNEL Beneficial for weak digestion. Used in gripe water, it can reduce colic, griping and wind. Also beneficial for acid ingestion, flatulence, hangovers, eye problems and travel sickness.

FEVERFEW Has been found to help with headaches, migraines, joint pains and period pains. The leaves make a good insect repellent, and in cases of insect bites or stings application of the tea can reduce swelling or pain.

GARLIC Another wonder herb, it was used during the war as a dressing for wounds prior to the discovery of antibiotics. It has numerous benefits for acne, digestive infections, candidiasis, warts, shingles, gum problems, sore throats and chest infections and can lower blood sugar and cholesterol levels. For earache break open a garlic capsule, use the contents to soak a small piece of cotton wool and place in the ear. Garlic can also be taken alongside antibiotics to reduce their side effects.

GINGER A natural intestinal antiseptic, beneficial for stomach conditions, nausea and morning sickness. Also an excellent herb for colds when crushed and used in combination with crushed garlic root.

GINGKO BILOBA Beneficial in opening up the cerebral blood flow, keeping mental faculties alert and helping memory. Trials have shown that Alzheimer's disease can be retarded with its use. Also beneficial for high blood pressure and tinnitus. Research has also shown that gingkolide, a primary constituent of gingko, has been effective in the treatment of irregular heartbeat. The leaves have been used for haemorrhoids, varicose veins and leg ulcers. As it generally improves nutrition to the brain, it can help guard against strokes. However, in cases of Alzheimer's disease and stroke, if a patient is on prescribed medication this should be taken into account as there is a possibility that gingko could interfere with the benefits. It is a best-selling herb in Germany.

GINSENG A wonderful tonic that has been used in China for over 5,000 years. Korean or Chinese ginseng replenishes spleen and lung energy and strengthens the immune system. Siberian ginseng is useful for short-term stressful events such as moving house. Astronauts are now being given Siberian ginseng to help them cope with the stress of being in outer space. It is advisable to avoid coffee when taking ginseng.

LEMON Anti-inflammatory, cooling, astringent, alkalizes the body and is beneficial to the liver and stomach.

LIMEFLOWERS Sedative and tranquillizing, it can help stress, tension, headaches, colds, flu, palpitations, anxiety and insomnia and can lower blood pressure. As it is rich in rutin, it can also help circulation and varicose veins.

LIQUORICE A wonder tonic and detoxifier, beneficial to the stomach as it soothes the mucous membranes, limiting acid production and preventing ulceration. It is also anti-inflammatory and can benefit arthritic conditions.

MARIGOLD (calendula) Used mainly as an ointment, it helps red sore skin, rashes (including nappy rash), sore nipples and sun burn.

MILK THISTLE Very beneficial for any liver disfunction such as hepatitis, jaundice, alcoholism, cirrhosis and gallstones. It also increases the body's ability to detoxify. Anyone taking highly toxic medication such as chemotherapy could benefit from taking milk thistle. For general use it is advisable to not take it at the same time as food.

NETTLE Contains large amounts of iron and vitamin C. Heals wounds and stops bleeding, is good for heavy menstrual bleeding. It is also anti-allergenic, a good skin herb and helps urticaria. The roots are thought to help prostate problems.

PASSIONFLOWER (*Passiflora*) Mildly sedative, it is good for anxiety, poor sleep, headaches, migraines and shock.

PEPPERMINT Beneficial for a number of digestive ailments such as indigestion, stomach cramps and acid reflex, bloating, travel sickness, diarrhoea and flatulence. It is also good for headaches and hangovers. It is best taken in tea form.

RASPBERRY LEAF An effective uterine tonic used in preparation for childbirth during the last three months of pregnancy, especially in combination with black cohash. Raspberry leaf is also useful for diarrhoea, sore throats and mouth ulcers because of its astringent effects.

RED CLOVER Mainly used for skin complaints such as eczema and psoriasis because of its cleansing and diuretic properties. It is also thought to have oestrogenic effects.

ROSEMARY Has a very uplifting and tonic effect. Stimulates mental activity and raises the spirits. The herb and the essential oil have completely different healing abilities. As a herb rosemary nourishes the adrenal glands, and used in conjunction with vervain it is beneficial for depression. It is also good for the hair. Rosemary should be avoided in cases of severe high blood pressure.

SAGE An oestrogenic, it has been known to help in menopausal conditions by reducing hot flushes and osteoporosis. It should be avoided during pregnancy as it can reduce breast milk production. Also an antiseptic herb, it is useful as a gargle for sore throats, mouth ulcers, insect bites and stings. It is good for digestion and can alleviate nervous sweating.

ST JOHN'S WORT Anti-inflammatory, astringent and a restorative tonic for the nervous system, relieving conditions such as sciatica, neuralgia, nervous exhaustion and depression.

VALERIAN A very relaxing and calming herb which benefits insomnia, muscle pain and tension, headaches, migraine and PMT. It is often combined with hops in sleep-inducing remedies, but sometimes hops can cause depression. It is beneficial for period pains when combined with cramp bark. It is important to start off with a small dose, such as half a teaspoon of tincture or one tablet or capsule, and then increase until the dose feels right for your personal needs.

VERVAIN Used widely in France as a digestive tonic, beneficial for liver and gallbladder conditions. It can innovate the heart by slowing its rate and can also counter the effects of stress.

CULINARY HERBS

There are also a few herbs used in the kitchen which have therapeutic benefits.

BASIL Good for the nervous system, and for digestion, and as a general tonic.

BAY Stimulates digestion.

BEETROOT Beneficial for anaemia as it is rich in iron.

CAYENNE Good for chilblains as it increases circulation. Use in moderation.

CINNAMON Taken as a tea it is beneficial for colds.

CLOVES Very good for toothache: chew a clove or apply clove oil to the affected tooth.

CORIANDER Beneficial for urinary tract infections and for generally strengthening the urinary system.

DILL Relieves flatulence and griping; often found in gripe water.

MINT Like peppermint, garden mint can aid digestion.

OREGANO Can relieve the symptoms of colds and coughs when used as an infusion. It can also aid digestion.

PARSLEY Contains high sources of vitamins and minerals, especially vitamin C and iron. Beneficial for arthritis and cystitis. When chewed, it makes a good breath freshener.

THYME An antiseptic and expectorant. Infusion is good for catarrh and chesty coughs.

USING HERBS

DECOCTIONS Use for roots, barks and some berries. Either grind into a powder or use 1 teaspoon to a cup of boiling water. Stir, cover and leave to stand for 5–10 minutes. Strain before drinking. Alternatively use 25g/1oz of root, bark or berries to 0.75 litre/1½pints of just-boiled water and simmer for 15 minutes in a saucepan. This will make 3 cups and can be kept for up to two days in a refrigerator.
Daily Dosage
Adults 1 cup two or three times.
Children up to one year One-tenth of the adult dosage.
Children of one to six years One-third of the adult dosage.
The elderly (over 70) 1–2 cups.

COMPRESSES Soak a piece of lint or a thin flannel in an infusion and apply to sore.or painful area.

TEAS Use a small handful of the fresh herb or 1 teaspoon of the dried herb to a cup of water just off the boil. To make three cups use 25g/1oz to 0.5 litre/17½fl oz of water. Make in a teapot or covered cup – cups with lids are available in most Chinese shops. Stir and leave to stand for 5–10 minutes, then strain and drink while hot. Any left-over tea can be drunk cold.
Daily Dosage
Adults 1 cup two to four times.
Children of up to one year One-tenth of the adult dosage.
Children of one to six years One-third of the adult dosage.
Children of six to 12 years Half the adult dosage.
The elderly (over 70) 2–3 cups.

TINCTURES Purchase from a herbalist or health-food shop. Do not combine them with other herbs as this diminishes their efficacy. Commercial tinctures are usually based in ethyl alcohol as a preservative and can last for up to two years. However, in cases of liver inflammation, pregnancy, reformed alcoholism or children it is best to add a small amount 25–50ml/¾–1¾fl oz of boiling water to the tincture dose and allow it to cool before taking. This will dissolve the alcohol.
Daily Dosage
Adults 1–2 teaspoons twice daily diluted in water. A little fruit juice can be added for taste.
Children As a rule children are given infusions rather than tinctures because the latter contain 45 per cent alcohol.
The elderly (over 70) 1–2 teaspoons as appropriate.

Consulting a Herbalist

Although most herbs are available over the counter, it is advisable when treating long-term or more serious problems to consult a herbal practitioner. The first consultation usually takes about an hour as the practitioner needs to look into the patient's medical history and generally enquire about diet, allergies, family medical history, stress, general lifestyle and any illness which currently exists. The herbalist will then make up a prescription in the form of a tincture, capsules, cream or the dried herbs themselves. Subsequent appointments usually last around 20–30 minutes and the herbal medication may be altered according to the condition of the patient.

It is important to inform your practitioner if you are taking any orthodox medication as there may be an incompatibility with some of the herbs. It is also important to inform the practitioner of any specific health problems such as liver and kidney disease, or if you are pregnant.

In the UK training to become a herbalist entails an intensive four- or five-year course. The National Institute of Medical Herbalists was founded in 1864 and qualified members use the initials MNIMH or FNIMH after their names. A list of qualified practitioners is available from the Institute (see page 219).

The power of herbs is boundless but, as with any remedy or treatment, the healing process must be a two-way course of development. Patients must take responsibility for their own health by improving their diet and lifestyle and always complete the prescribed course of treatment.

With mortality an inevitable part of life, the important thing is to grow old gracefully but realistically. Better health comes from a positive attitude of mind, acquiring enough sleep, taking sufficient exercise and eating a well-managed diet. My hope is that this book will have given you the information and advice you need to help you make the necessary choices for a healthier, happier future, both in body and soul. As Hippocrates said a couple of thousand years ago, 'A wise man ought to realize that health is his most valuable possession' – and, of course, he meant that women should too.

USEFUL ADDRESSES

CHAPTER 1

Help the Aged
St James' Walk
London EC1R 0BE
Tel: 0171-253 0253

The Soil Association
86 Colston Street
Bristol BS1 5BB
Tel: 0117-929 0661
Fax: 0117-925 2504

Osteoporosis Society
PO Box 10, Radstock
Bath
Avon BA3 3YB
Tel: 01761-432472

Arthritis Care
18 Stephenson Way
London NW1 2HD
Tel: 0171-916 1500

Arthritic Association (aims to help
through natural methods)
2 Hyde Gardens
Eastbourne
Sussex BN21 4PN

Alzheimer's Disease Society
2nd Floor, Gordon House
10 Greencoat Place
London SW1 1PH
Tel: 0171-306 0606

Multiple Sclerosis Society of Great
Britain and Northern Ireland
25 Effie Road
London SW6 1EE
Tel: 0171-610 7171

Parkinson's Disease Association
12 Upper Woburn Place
London WC1H 0EP
Tel: 0171-383 3513

The British Thyroid Foundation
PO Box HP22
Leeds
Yorkshire LS6 3RT

British Diabetic Association
10 Queen Anne Street
London W1M 0BD
Tel: 0171-323 1531

ME Association
Stanhope House, High Street
Stanford-le-Hope
Essex SS17 OHA
Tel: 01375-642466

National AIDS Helpline
Tel: 0800 567123

Cancer Relief Macmillan Fund
15 Britten Street
London SW3 3TZ
Tel: 0171-353 7811

Bristol Cancer Help Centre
Grove House,
Clifton
Bristol BS8 4PG
Tel: 0117-980 9500
Fax: 0117-923 9184

The British Heart Foundation
14 Fitzhardinge Street
London W1H 4DH
Tel: 0171-935 0185

The Stroke Association
CHSA House, Whitecross Street
London EC1Y
Tel: 0171-490 7999

Endometriosis Society Charity
5 Artillery Row
London SW1P 1RL
Tel: 0171-222 2776

Pre-Menstrual Tension Advisory
Service
PO Box 268, Hove
East Sussex BN3 1R3

Women's Health
52-54 Featherstone Street
London EC1Y 8RT
Tel: 0171-251 6580

Wellbeing (the only charity to fund
research into womens health)
27 Sussex Place
London NW1 4SP
Tel: 0171-262 5337

The Herpes Association
41 North Road
London N7 9DP
Tel: 0171-609 9061

Breast Care Campaign
1 St Mary Abbots Place
London W8 6LS
Tel: 0171-371 1510

Amarant Trust (HRT)
Grant House, 56–60 St John Street
London EC1M 4DT
Tel: 0171-490 1644

The Psoriasis Association
Milton House, 7 Milton Street
Northampton NN2 7JG
Tel: 01604-711129

National Eczema Society
163 Eversholt Street
London NW1 1BU
Tel: 0171-388 4097

International Glaucoma Association
(Mrs B Wright)
c/o Kings College Hospital
Denmark Hill
London SE5 9RS
Tel: 0171-737 3265

Trayner Pinhole Glasses
Sturminster Newton (GL)
Dorset DT10 1EJ

Royal National Institute for the Blind
(RNIB)
224 Great Portland Street
London W1N 6AA
Tel: 0171-388 1266

The Bates Association of GB
(Enclose SAE for details)
PO Box 25,
Shoreham by Sea
West Sussex BN43 6ZF

Royal National Institute for the Deaf
(RNID)
105 Gower Street
London WC1E 6AH
0171-387 8033

CHAPTER 2
Miscarriage Association
c/o Clayton Hospital
Northgate, Wakefield
West Yorkshire WF1 3JS
Tel: 01924-200799

Association of Post Natal Illness
25 Jerden Place
London SW6 1BE
Tel: 0171-386 0868

Relate – National Marriage
Guidance
Herbert Gray College
Little Church Street
Rugby
Warwickshire CN21 3AP
Tel: 01788-573241

Release (drug-related problems)
388 Old Street
London EC1V 9LT

Association of Retired Persons
Greencoat House
London SW1P 1DZ
Tel: 0171-895 8880

Seasonal Affective Disorder
Association
PO Box 989
London SW7 2PZ
Tel: 01903-814942

Sivananda Yoga Vedanta Centre
51 Felsham Road
London SW15 1AZ
Tel: 0181-780 0160

The Floatation Tank Association
South London Natural Health
Association
7A Clapham Common Southside
London SW4 7AA
Tel:0171-627 4962

National Family Meditation
Tavistock Place
London WC1H 9SN
Tel: 0171-383 5993

National Register of
Psychotherapists and
Hypnotherapists
12 Cross Streeet
Nelson
Lancashire
Tel: 01282-699378

British Association for Autogenic
Training and Therapy
18 Holtsmere Close
Watford
Hertfordshire WD2 6NG

Body Stress Release
Contact: Peter Van Minnen
Tel: 01959-565926/0171-379 7662

The Bach Centre
Mount Vernon
Sotwell, Wallingford
Oxon OX10 0PZ
Tel: 01491-834678

Nelsons Pharmacy
73 Duke Street
London W1M 6BY
Tel: 0171-495 2404

CHAPTER 3
British Chiropractic Association
Premier House
10 Greycoat Place
London SW1P 1SB
Tel: 01734-757557

Institute for Complementary
Medicine
PO Box 194
London SE16 1QZ
Tel: 0171-237 5765

International Federation of
Aromatherapists
Stamford House
2–4 Chiswick High Road
London W4 1TH
Tel: 0181-742 2606

The Shiatsu Society
5 Foxcote
Wokingham
Berkshire RG11 3PG

MLD UK
8 Wittenham Lane
Dorchester-on-Thames
Oxfordshire X10 7JW

Association of Ayurvedic
Practitioners
50 Penywern Road
London SW5 9SX
Tel: 0171-370 2255

Association of Reflexologists
27 Old Gloucester Street
London WC1N 3XX
Tel: 01892-512612

British Acupuncture Association
34 Alderney Street
London SW1V 4EU
Tel: 0171-834 1012

British Naturopathic and
Osteopathic Association
6 Netherall Gardens
London NW3 5RR
Tel: 0171-435 7830

CHAPTER 4
The Exercise Asssociation
Unit 4 Angel Gate, City Road
London EC1V 2PT
Tel: 0171-278 0811

Gripmaster Stockists
Lyon Equipment Ltd
Rise Hill Mill
Dent, Sedbergh
Cumbria LA10 5QL
Tel: 015396-25493

Therapeutic Putty
John Bell and Croyden
0171-935 5555

Lotte Berk Studio
29 Manchester Street
London W1
Tel: 0171-935 8905

Alexander Technique
20 London House
266 Fulham Road
London SW10 9EL
Tel: 0171 351 0828

Pilates Teachers Association
17 Queensberry Mews West
London SW7 2DY
Tel: 0171-581 7041
Fax: 0171-581 2286

The School of T'ai Chi Chuan
5 Tavistock Place
London WC1H 9SS

CHAPTER 5
The Vegan Society
Donald Watson House
7 Battle Road
St Leonard-on-Sea
East Sussex TN37 7AA
Tel: 01424-427393

Association of Systematic
Kinesiology – (Registered Charity)
Dunham Road, Altricham
Cheshire WA4 4QG
Tel: 0161-928 0793

British Allergy Foundation
St Bartholomew's Hospital
West Smithfield
London EC1A 7BE
Tel: 0171-600 6127

National Institute of Herbal Medicine
9 Palace Gate,
Exeter
Devon EX1 1JA

REFERENCES

CHAPTER 1
Age Erasers (Rodale Press, 1994, USA) 90, 91, 92, passim

'Cervical Smears' and 'Malula Degeneration' *Reader's Digest Good Health Fact Book* (Reader's Digest Association Ltd, 1991) 164, 427

Reader's Digest Good Health Fact Book (Reader's Digest Association Ltd, 1991)

Bawden, F 'HRT – The Myths Exploded' *What Doctors Don't Tell You* (Wallace Press) vol 4, no 9, 2

'Research into Ageing' *You and Your Health Magazine* (November 1995)

'The Air We Breathe' *Reader's Digest Good Health Fact Book* (Reader's Digest Association Ltd, 1991) 302-307

Carter, R 'Talking about Incontinence' *Top Santé Magazine* (September 1994) 42, 43

Curtis, S & Fraser, R *Natural Healing for Women* (Pandora Press, 1991) 171, 173

Earle, L *Healthy Menopause* (Boxtree Ltd, 1995) 11–24

Flemin, J E 'Studying the Ageing Process' *Complementary Medicine Magazine*

Forrest, N H et al *Paper on Boron* (United States Department of Agriculture, 1987, USA)

Graham, J *Multiple Sclerosis: a self help guide* (HarperCollins, 1996)

Greer, R & Woodward Dr R *Anti-oxidant Nutrition* (Souvenir Press Ltd, 1995) 19

Herzberg, E I 'Cancer - The Power of Hope' *Here's Health Magazine* (March 1996) 25, 27

Kyrias, M 'Free Radicals and Ageing' *Care of the Elderly* (July 1994) 260, 262

Mervin, L *Stomach Ulcers and Acidity* (Thorsons, 1990)

Neil, K *Balancing Hormones Naturally* (ION Press, 1994) 30–34

Reader's Digest Family Guide to Alternative Medicine (Reader's Digest Association, 1991) 126, 279

Smart, F (with Prof S Campbell) *Fibroids* (Thorsons, 1993) 25, 26

Smith, T (ed) 'Menopause and Menorrhagia' *The British Medical Association Complete Family Health Encyclopaedia* (Dorling Kindersley, 1990) 676

Spirduso, W *Physical Dimension of Ageing* (Human Kinetics Publishers, 1995, USA) 6, 20

Stewart, Dr A & Maryon *Beat IBS through Diet* (Vermillion, 1994) 32, 81

Stewart, M *Beat the Menopause without HRT* (Headline Book Publishing, 1995) 3–17, 34–52

The Wellcome Trust *Diving into the Gene Pool* (Medical Research Council, 1995)

Werbach, Dr M R *Healing through Nutrition* (Thorsons, 1995) 174,175

CHAPTERS 2 and 3
Gaia, *The Book of Yoga* (Ebury Press, 1983)

Glasstock, G & Gressor, M *Coping with Loss and Grief* (Robinsons Publishing Ltd, 1995) 78–85

MacDonald, H 'Don't be SAD' *Here's Health Magazine* (December 1995) 30, 31, 32

CHAPTER 4
Buzan, T *Use Your Head* (BBC Books, 1989)

Carter, A E *The Miracles of Rebound Exercise* (Snohomish Publishing Co, 1979, USA)

Friedman, P & Eisen, G *The Pilates Method of Mental and Physical Conditioning* (Warner Books, 1980, USA)

Gordon, N F *Arthritis: Your Complete Exercise Guide* (Human Kinetics Publishers, 1993, USA)

Gordon, N F *Stroke: Your Complete Exercise Guide* (Human Kinetics Publishers, 1993, USA)

Leon, A S et al 'Use it or Lose it: Leisure-time Physical Activity Levels and Risk of Coronary Heart Disease and Death' *Journal of American Medical Association* (1987) vol 258, 2388–2395

Raglin, G S 'Exercise and Mental Health - Beneficial and Detrimental Effects' *Sports Medicine* (1990) vol 9, 323–329

Samples P 'Exercise Encouraged for People with Arthritis' *Physician and Sports Medicine* (1990) vol 18,123-126

Tangeman, P T et al 'Rehabilitation of Chronic Stroke Patients: Changes of Functional Performance' *Archives of Physical Medicine and Rehabilitation* (1990) 876–880

CHAPTER 5
'The Allergy Revolution' *Here's Health Magazine* (March 1996) 64

'Vegetarianism' *Health Guardian* (March/April 1996)

Appleton, N *Lick the Sugar Habit* (Avery Publishing, 1988, USA) 4, 15

Ester, C *Nutrition News* (1991) vol 14, 3

Erasmus, U *Fats that Heal, Fats that Kill* (Alive Books, 1995, USA)

Foods That Heal Foods That Harm (Reader's Digest Association Ltd, 1996) 150–153

Griggs, B 'Aloe, Aloe' *Country Living Magazine* (February/March) 122, 124

Kenton, L *The Joy of Beauty* (Arrow Books, 1983) 71

Mindell, E *The Anti-Ageing Bible* (Souvenir Press Ltd, 1995) 211

Noakes, B 'The Fats of Life' *Here's Health Magazine* (November 1995) 50

Porter, S 'Caffeine and Your Body' *Which Way to Health Magazine* (October 1995) 168–169

Setniker, I et al 'Pharmacokinetics of Glucosamine in the Dog and Man' *Arzneimittelforschung* (1991) vol 36, no 2, 729–736

Ursell, A 'Are You a Salt Fiend?' *Here's Health Magazine* (November 1995) 45

Ursell, A 'The Caffeine Controversy' *Here's Health Magazine* (October 1995) 49

Wheater, C *The Juicing Detox Diet* (Thorsons, 1993)

Wunderlich, R C Jr MD *Sugar and Your Health* (Good Health Publications, 1982, USA) 37

INDEX

Index